T0106901

I KNOW HOW TO LOSE WEIGHT, SO WHY CAN'T I KEEP IT OFF?

I KNOW HOW TO LOSE WEIGHT, SO WHY CAN'T I KEEP IT OFF?

NICK HALL, PhD

MEDIA

MEDIA

Published 2019 by Gildan Media LLC
aka G&D Media
www.GanddMedia.com

FIRST EDITION 2019

Front Cover design by David Rheinhardt of Pyrographx

Interior design by Meghan Day Healey of Story Horse, LLC

Library of Congress Cataloging-in-Publication Data is available upon request

ISBN: 978-1-7225-0014-6

10   9   8   7   6   5   4   3   2   1

Contents

Introduction

Mary had always had a problem with her weight. Even in middle school, she was heavier than the other girls despite being careful about what she ate. Her mother was a Registered Dietician so made sure her daughter had well balanced and nutritious meals. She was on the swim and track teams for all four years of high school, yet Mary still was heavier than she wanted to be. But despite her personal preference for a certain appearance, was she really unhealthy? Probably not!

Many children and adults struggle needlessly with their weight. When defining optimal health, one size does not fit all despite cultural pressure to squeeze everyone into the smallest dress size possible. Whether monitoring body weight, body mass index, waist to hip ratio, or percent body fat, the quest always seems to be for less. Before continuing with this program, ask yourself these three questions to decide if you really need to be worried about your weight:

1. Am I comfortable with my current body weight?
2. Am I in good cardiovascular health?
3. Am I able to maintain the weight acceptable to me without constant dieting?
4. Am I able to do all the things I want to?

If your answer to each of those questions is, YES, then there's really no need to do anything except use the advice in this program to maintain the status quo.

I *know* I should lose weight so why don't I?

In this book, we'll explore why this question is so common among all of us "mere mortals" who have struggled with weight issues throughout our lives. And we'll explore the answer to this question—with scientific research on exactly why it is that most people cannot keep those extra pounds off. But, best of all, I'll give you specific scientifically proven steps that you can take to keep those pounds off, and eradicate this question from your consciousness once and for all!

Let's consider the attitude of the British singing sensation, Adele Adkins. Adele was cruelly ridiculed by Joan Rivers who, on the David Letterman Show remarked that Adele should have named her hit song *Rolling in the Deep Fried Chicken.* That's because in the eyes of some, she didn't conform to the norm. But Adele saw things from a very different, and I might add healthy perspective when she was interviewed for the February 2012 edition of People Magazine. "I've never wanted to look like models on the cover of magazines. I represent the majority of women and I'm very proud of that," she declared.

There's also the matter of the Obesity Paradox; the research finding published in the medical journal, Mayo Clinic Proceedings, revealing that obesity can be correlated with a significant reduction in all-cause mortality. Others showed that an important factor explaining the paradox is the amount of lean body mass compared with fat. This should not be taken as justification to tear up your gym membership, and snack on junk food while setting up residence on your couch. The Obesity Paradox applies to only those individuals who fall into a unique category of having a large amount of lean tissue, which is muscle. For those without this lean tissue, heart disease, musculoskeletal disorders, and type II diabetes are just some of the health consequences of carry excessive body weight.

Factors Affecting Weight Loss

I bring this up because losing weight is not a simple matter of dieting or burning excess calories through more exercise. There are many factors involved including your DNA.

Your genetic blueprint sets the stage for everything, including body weight. But genes predict probability, not causality. Having a gene associated with a particular trait is no guarantee you'll acquire it. There are factors capable of activating and deactivating genes. These are known as epigenetic factors. Age and physical characteristics such as bone mass are important as well. But something that is generating a great deal of scientific inquiry is the role of bacteria. Not the kind that trigger infection. Rather, we are looking at the bacteria that live inside us as part of what is called the microbiome. This emerging research suggests that providing for a healthy mix of beneficial bacteria may also need to be incorporated into a successful weight loss equation. There's one more very important factor that needs to be dealt with—stress. Emotional upheaval can trigger changes in your brain chemistry driving a craving for carbohydrate and fat laden foods. That's why the expression, 'emotional eating' is used to describe why people under stress may turn to so called comfort foods.

The human brain, despite its enormous complexity, has really just one function; to keep us alive. We approach those things likely to promote our survival and avoid those things that threaten it. Many of the integral processes operate below the conscious radar. For example, we breathe, our heart keeps beating, and critical chemicals are maintained at just the right level without our conscious awareness of the complex biological machinery operating beneath the skin. But when all the biochemistry is stripped away, the process is really quite straightforward. Each system has a means by which to regulate itself through a system of feed-back pathways. When supply is sufficient, production ceases. When more is needed, the assembly line is cranked up. Our behavior is subject to the same basic rules. When we perceive a threat to our wellbeing, we take steps to avoid the potentially harmful circumstances. In contrast, when circumstances are promoting our well-being, we engage in behaviors to get more. Yes, it's that simple. The brain is essentially an organ that secretes behavior. We approach or we avoid. And we decide which is appropriate depending upon which emotion is in place. Positive emotions such as joy and love motivate us to seek more, while negative emotions such as disgust and sadness motivate us to seek less. This program will explore the start and stop signals that regulate eating behavior.

All behavior is governed by the same set of rules. There has to be an initial signal that sets in motion a specific response, which ultimately adjusts the signal. Using the example of eating, the signal is the sensation of hunger, the response is consumption of food, and then as the stomach fills, messages arrive in the brain to turn the signal off. However, in the interest of efficiency, this otherwise straightforward process can sometimes take a short cut. Instead of waiting for hunger to arise, other things may acquire the ability to trigger the consumption of food. You may fall into the routine of eating at the same time of day, because that's when lunch is scheduled. Eventually, you eat not because you're hungry, but because the response of eating has become entrained to the time of day. Or you may eat in response to activity.

Have you ever visited the zoo shortly before feeding time? If so, you've watched the big cats pace back and forth from one end of their enclosure to the other. The monkeys leapt from one object to another, while the birds flew around their exhibit. Even though the routine included the delivery of food to their cage, they became active prior to the food's arrival in response to other environmental cues. In response to a variety of cues, they ostensibly began to forage for food. Not only do all animals, including humans, become more active before scheduled mealtimes, but there are episodic bursts in the levels of cortisol, the energy producing steroid which makes sure your tissues have the required fuel to engage in the quest for food. After doing this repeatedly, the activity becomes so closely aligned with eating that it eventually has the ability to replace hunger as a signal to eat. This works in other ways as well.

Boredom drives some people to eat as a means by which to offset monotony. Eating becomes the activity the person is seeking to achieve some balance in their life. The result is eating when food is not needed, which results in extra calories, which will be stored as fat. It doesn't matter whether those calories are in the form of carbohydrate, fat, or protein; if you don't need them you will store them. That's why strategies for coping with stress, whether due to anxiety or boredom, must be a part of any body weight management strategy.

This same basic process of a stimulus leading to a response can also take place well below the conscious radar. Psychoneuroimmunology is the study of how the brain, emotions and behavior can interface with the immune system, which we need to fight infection and cancer. While the role of emotions in modulating disease has a long and hallowed history dating to the observations of ancient Greek physicians, it was not until Drs. Robert Ader and Nicholas Cohen at the University of Rochester demonstrated that the immune system could respond to unrelated cues that the field became the subject of serious scientific inquiry. These two scientists administered a drug that temporarily reduced the number of disease fighting white cells in laboratory mice. At the same time, the animals were allowed to taste water flavored with saccharin. Saccharine is an artificial sweetener that does nothing to the immune system. However, after pairing the sweet flavor with the drug, just the taste was capable of reducing the white cell count. That experiment has now been repeated in many clinical contexts included in the study of cancer and autoimmune disease. This groundbreaking experiment launched the field of Psychoneuroimmunology. It also affirmed that cues with no direct association with a particular biological system, could acquire that ability through an automatic learning process call Classical Conditioning. This principal had been demonstrated decades earlier when Ivan Pavlov, while studying dogs, triggered salivation by simply ringing a bell, which had previously been paired with the sight and smell of food.

A man obviously searching for something under a street light was asked by a stranger what he was looking for. "My keys" was the answer. "Is this where you lost them?" the stranger asked? "No. I lost them over there." Then why aren't you looking over there?" "Because there's more light over here!" That's the mistake made by many people attempting to lose weight. They take steps to change the obvious behavior they associate with food. They start with their appetite or hunger signals, which everyone knows are associated with the desire to eat. However, the actual cause of overeating may have no obvious connection to food at all. It may be in the dark regions of your understanding. Overlooking the role of unrelated cues is often the reason sustaining a weight management program can be so difficult. Just about anything has the potential ability to trigger eating as a result of the automatic learning process called Classical Conditioning.

Here's the good news. By definition, those things we do automatically as a result of conditioning can be de-conditioned. But only if you know what the trigger is. Once you become consciously aware of what causes the desire to eat, it's a matter of experiencing the trigger then making sure the normal response does not occur. It may take a lot of will-power, but once you understand why it's important to do so, you will be more likely to succeed. Eventually, the urge to eat in response to these conditioned cues will go away. You've succeeded in breaking the unhealthy habit; however, you'll still have to contend with other biological drives, including some occurring deep within your brain.

This book will provide you with an understanding of how the brain drives us to seek fat or carbohydrates when those foods are likely to promote survival. It will include a discussion of why stress and the associated emotions are an important cue in stimulating health-destructive eating behavior, as well as ways you can reduce or even stop the desire to eat before it arises. However, the one thing it can't do is provide you with the motivation to change. That is entirely in your hands. What I will do is explain the normal processes of appetite regulation along with the things you can do to take control. In this way, I can instill in you a sense of optimism that you will be successful.

What Do I Want To Achieve?

D o you want to lose weight? "Of course", you might reply. "Why else would I have purchased this book?" What I really mean is have you taken the time to reflect upon what is involved? Let's begin that process now. Start with your long-term objective, which should not be to lose weight. Your ultimate goal should be something highly personal, not simply to please someone else. If that happens, all well and good, however, it should not be your primary objective. As you reflect upon your ultimate objective, make sure it meets the following criteria:

1. It must be attainable.
2. It must be measurable.
3. It mustn't conflict with other important goals you may have.
4. It must be dependent upon losing weight.
5. It must be personal.

Here are some suggestions:
- I want to enjoy dancing at my grandchild's wedding.
- I want to enjoy my favorite leisure activities well into retirement.
- I want to hike the length of the Appalachian Trail.

Achieving each of these goals is contingent upon achieving a healthful weight. Of course there are other things you would need to do as well, including exercise if you're going to accomplish the more physically demanding objectives. However, losing weight is not the goal. That's a necessary step, indeed an important part of the process, but it's not the main objective. If you focus on losing weight, you may quickly become frustrated and conclude your chosen approach can't work. That would be an erroneous and premature conclusion. Initially you may gain pounds as fat is lost, and muscle is gained. Muscle attracts water so is heavier than hydrophobic fat. You'll start to look and feel better, and experience more energy, but perceive yourself as a failure and give up if losing weight is your primary objective.

Perhaps these things I listed are not priorities for you, in which case think of something you have always dreamed about doing, and define that as your goal. But remember, it's got to be what intuitively feels right for you, not what you think is expected of you by associates or family members. You must also make a commitment to achieve your goal. This may be easier said than done. Unexpected setbacks may temporarily require your full attention. Therefore, take time to anticipate what is likely to happen that might prevent you from achieving your objective. If it is insurmountable, then how might you modify your goal so you can still achieve part of it? Always have a backup plan. It's OK to make modifications, but not to give up entirely unless there truly are extenuating circumstances. Doing the latter will simply reinforce your belief that you are a failure. Of course you'll be less likely to encounter setbacks if you heed the advice of Lord Baden Powell—*Be Prepared*.

Making a commitment to achieve any goal will entail the need to make sacrifices and to delaying gratification. Chances are, an unwillingness to recognize and then do these things may well be the reason you have been unsuccessful in the past. That's all going to change because you're going to anticipate setbacks before they happen and then incorporate into your protocol a means by which to keep them from becoming permanent. I'll begin by asking you to reflect upon previous attempts, if any, to get more healthy.

Have you tried to lose weight in the past? If so, what were the things that kept you from doing so?

Was it time constraints? *I don't have time to shop for the right foods, I work too many hours to exercise, or shopping for the right foods is inconvenient.*

Perhaps it was lack of knowledge? *I don't know what are healthy choices, my doctor never tells me to lose weight, or I lost the list of foods I should avoid and those I should eat.*

Maybe it was the environment? *I'm not the one who buys groceries, I live in a dangerous neighborhood so I can't exercise, or I am under too much stress at work.*

Or was it your attitude? *I can't stick to a strict diet, I don't like any of the foods that are good for me, or I hate exercise.*

Some people may express a reason that is not really the one holding them back. Indeed, it may be buried in their self-conscious or they just don't want to admit it to others. For example, the real reason for not taking steps to lose weight and achieve a state of optimal health may be one of the following:

- It's an excuse to avoid feelings of failure.
- It's a form of denial that poor health is a consequence of unhealthy eating.
- It's the consequence of depression, which saps the motivation to get healthy.
- It's the desire to avoid intimacy.

These are the reasons you must start by asking, *Do I want to lose weight*? If you're not ready, then starting prematurely will inevitable result in failure making it less likely you'll be successful at another time. You'll conclude, *I've tried it before and it doesn't work*!

Once you've identified your ultimate objective, ask these questions:

- Is my goal realistic? Is it something I can actually achieve? I'm 67 and weigh 150 pounds. Stating my goal of being hired as a defensive back for a professional football team would be unrealistic. However, being competitive on a Masters Swim team would be a very realistic.

- Is it my goal or someone else's? Are you being pressured by an employer or family member to achieve a goal, or is it really yours?

- Is my goal stated concisely and in a positive way? For example, instead of, *I want to avoid being bed ridden* state it as, *I want to be active when I retire.*

- Is my goal compatible with my values and beliefs? Even though I described it as a goal, walking the entire Appalachian Trail as a through-hiker would not be appropriate for someone who values time with family. Of course it could be done in segments or even better, take the family with you. I have two good friends who sailed around the world, yet valued time with their children and grandchildren. They would complete a segment, take time off to fly back to America to be with family, and then continue the voyage when they were ready. It took them 20 years to complete the circumnavigation! By modifying their goal, they succeeded without compromising what they valued most—time with their children and grandchildren without missing a single milestone as they grew into young adulthood. And what an inspiration they are to the next generation!

- *What am I willing to give up to achieve my goal?* That's all part of anticipating setbacks along the way. You may not have to compromise at all. But thinking it through is a crucial part of deciding, am I ready to start?

Reasons for Failure

The reason you might have been unsuccessful in the past is because of the approach you took to losing weight. Reflect upon which of the following you might have done either alone or in combination.

- Foregoing breakfast, lunch or dinner.
- Cutting back on or eliminating fat or carbohydrates.
- Increasing the amount or intensity of exercise.
- Cutting out unhealthy snacks and soda.
- Taking prescription or over the counter drugs to lose weight.
- Purging yourself through laxatives or vomiting.

Most of these strategies represent short-cuts to losing weight. Not only that, anytime you restrict your intake of food, whether by category or amount, you run the risk of becoming undernourished unless you take the time to learn what you have to do to take in the essential nutrients. Cutting back on macronutrients may not be healthy, and relying on any type of medication can lead to dependency as well as adverse side effects. Of course purging the body of food can alter your electrolyte and fluid balance, not to mention leaving you malnourished. Of the common strategies I just reviewed, the only two acceptable ones are increasing the amount or intensity of exercise, and cutting out unhealthy snacks and soda. Before continuing, you need to be aware of the essentials you must do no matter what. Chances are when consuming more food than you need, even though you aren't paying particular attention to the amount of vitamins and minerals in your meals, you're still getting what you need. But when you start restricting your dietary intake, you run the risk of leaving some critically needed ingredients out.

Any dietary approach that is going to be successful must be systemic. By that I mean you should realize the ultimate objective is to achieve a state of optimal health, which requires nutrients that will benefit the heart, brain, immune system along with all the other physiological processes we depend upon for good health. That necessitates doing a number of things simultaneously. For example, adhering to a regular exercise program, obtaining the amount and type of sleep you need, and taking steps to reduce the stress in your life. Each of these can impact your appetite and so ignoring them will lead to failure. Other obstacles are part of what the US Department of Disease Prevention and Health Promotion refers to as the obesogenic environment, which for many people includes an overabundance of stress, and convenient access to energy dense, but nutrient poor foods.

Obstacles to Success

This book will begin with the important task of defining your goal and in a way you are likely to achieve it. I'll then describe a two-step process whereby you will significantly increase your chances of success. However, before taking pro-active steps to achieve an optimal body weight, you need to eliminate or at least minimize the obstacles. The biggest one? Stress!

Stress

Many people experience chronic stress, which will increase significantly the ingestion and storage of food. There are several reasons for this. First, during times of emotional upheaval, we need more energy to fuel the fight/flight response. That doesn't necessarily mean you are in a dire situation. Worrying may cause a slight increase in heart rate as you contemplate your circumstances. Energy is required to fuel that increase, along with other perhaps subtle biological events including the production of chemicals capable of changing your metabolism and altering your mood, sleep habits, and ability to concentrate.

It begins with the perception of a potential threat. This in turn will trigger the production of a brain chemical called corticotropin releasing hormone (CRH) inside the part of the brain that monitors the environment 24/7. It's called the amygdala and can be thought of as the brain's office of homeland security. Its job is to connect the dots and when a threat is perceived, give rise to the emotion of fear. Studies have shown that this can happen below the conscious radar. When a person is shown a picture of something they are deathly afraid of, perhaps a coiled rattlesnake, they respond with an anxious plea to take the picture away as their heart rate increases. However, when the picture is cut into more than a hundred pieces of random shapes and sizes, and then glued to a board of the same size as the original, they shrug and ask, "What's that supposed to be?" as they examine the jumbled image. There's no conscious recognition, however, their heart rate increases in response to the subconscious threat. It all happens in the amygdala, which plays an important role in what is called intuition.

The word 'emotion' shares the same root as 'motivate'. That's what emotions do. They motivate us to approach those things associated with positive emotions such as love and happiness, but to avoid those things associated with negative emotions, such as fear and sadness. That's one of the jobs of corticotropin releasing hormone. It will trigger increased alertness, which in excess might be called anxiety. It also lowers the levels of the neurotransmitter capable of regulating both mood and sleep, called serotonin. Of course if you are about to engage in physical action, which is quite likely when a threat in pending, you want to be alert and not sleepy. You also want to eat foods capable of being converted very quickly into energy. The best food for this is carbohydrate, and that's what the stress-induced drop in serotonin will motivate you to do; crave carbohydrates. Carbohydrate is exactly what its name describes; hydrated carbon. It's nothing more than carbon attached to water, which makes it easy for them to be quickly absorbed through the cells lining the gut. Its entry is heralded by a rise in blood glucose, which the liver stores either as glycogen, or lets travel in the blood to the tissues that need it. Here's where things start to get interesting.

Carbohydrates, especially in the form of sugary dessert, taste really good. Indeed, it's the reward or hedonic properties of food that entice us to eat them. Stress makes food even more rewarding. Here's why. CRH stimulates the release of cortisol. Cortisol enables the body to produce glucose from protein just in case we can't get enough carbohydrate to fuel our response. It also makes food even more rewarding than it already is. Actually, it makes everything more rewarding by increasing the salience of pleasurable or compulsive activities. That's why people may go on a shopping spree, turn to drugs, or ingest more sugary and fatty foods than usual. Eating in excess purely for pleasure in the absence of hunger is called hedonic hyperphagia. That's what stress makes you do. No wonder fat and carbohydrate laden meals are sometimes categorized as comfort food. There's more.

The main stress hormone, cortisol, results in the storage of excess fat in the abdominal region. This growing population of fat cells then transmits chemical messages to the brain telling it to end the stress response. Not only that, but through a purely pleasure pathway, sugar water has been found to reduce the entire chemical stress response in laboratory experiments.

Does this happen outside the lab in the world we live in? Absolutely. When an infant is about to be vaccinated or circumcised, attending nurses will sometimes dip a pacifier into a container of sugar water or allow the child to lick a piece of candy just before the invasive procedure is carried out. When the anticipated scream becomes nothing more than a whimper, it's a pretty good indication that using pleasure as a way to reduce stress is not just a laboratory phenomenon, but one with clinical applications as well. So what does all this mean? During stress, we are drawn to eat foods capable of reducing the tension. In other words, when people turn to comfort foods, they are self-medicating. Virtually any stressful environment including work, home and/or school can trigger overeating.

This would not be a problem if stress were short-lived. During the stone-age, most stressors did not last very long. When your ancestral relative had an altercation with his neighbor, it would be resolved very quickly with one person emerging victorious and the other suffering defeat. That's not the way it is in today's world. There are some people who work in settings they hate. They can't stand their supervisor, despise their co-workers, and dread having to interact with clients. Just driving into the parking lot and entering the building can trigger anxiety. So why stay? Many people will answer, 'because I need the health benefits'. How ironic, yet true. The World Health Organization has identified stress as a factor in the etiology of more than half the diseases we experience. There are other reasons people remain in stressful jobs or toxic relationships. For example, they might be locked into a lucrative retirement plan. Or leaving may be too disruptive for family members. Of course there's also the possibility that jobs in their profession are limited so they have no choice but to remain.

Instead of eating a few energy dense meals during the short term crisis that will soon be resolved, the eating continues for an extended period when the stress continues. What would be a normal and beneficial response when measured in days or perhaps a few weeks becomes a major health problem when the emotional-eating continues for months or even years. That's why this program will explore several options for dealing with stress as a means by which to better manage body weight.

Emotional Eating

Stress gets blamed for everything. It seems that the shelves of bookstores and the words of self-proclaimed stress experts are filled with the advice that if you can somehow vanquish the stress in your life, your immune system, memory, and mood problems will vanish like a snowball on a hot stove. That is not true. Stress is not the cause of your physical and mental health problems and eliminating it will not necessarily be the answer to your health concerns. Stress creates an environment within your body making it easier for other things to do the dirty work. For example, infection is caused by viruses and bacteria. However, the chemistry of stress makes it more difficult for your immune system to ward of those microbes. Not only is stress not the direct problem, under the right circumstances, it's actually beneficial. Imagine how boring life would be if there were no uncertainty. Your health and well-being are comparable to a muscle. Wrap a broken arm or leg in a cast, and within a matter of days it will begin to atrophy. The muscle fibers need constant stress just to maintain them at their existing level. When an athlete wants to achieve a higher level of functioning, she doesn't lay on the couch and rest. She pushes herself even more until she emerges from a zone of discomfort at a new and enhanced level of strength and endurance. It's the same for every aspect of life and happiness. Stress is a stimulus for mental, physical and spiritual growth. However, it is during periods of recovery when that growth occurs. It is rare for a person to have too much stress; invariably the problem is a lack of recovery. For every action, there has to be an equal and opposite reaction. Even if you have world-class stress, as long as you balance it with world-class recovery, you will thrive. A well-documented consequence of an imbalance between stress and recovery is overeating, along with the deposition of fat in the abdominal or visceral area. Fat in that part of the body increases a person's risk for inflammatory disease, heart conditions, and cancer. Eating food in response to stress is referred to as emotional eating, and the types of foods people gravitate toward are called comfort foods. Stress is without question the major cause of overeating. Therefore, taking steps to reduce stress is imperative if a weight management program is to be successful. Failure to address this is probably the most common answer to the question, *I know how to lose weight, so why can't I keep it off*? That's why this next section will be devoted to the things you can do to achieve balance between stress and recovery.

Stress Management

In a previous section, I described the mechanism whereby stress can reduce brain levels of serotonin thereby paving the way to depression and carbohydrate craving. Let's tackle that problem first. It won't be easy because eating carbohydrate will ultimately be the solution. It will make you feel better, which will make the desire for it that more challenging to ignore. Studies have revealed that when a laboratory rat is fed sucrose or sugar water just before being exposed to a mild form of stress, the normal rise in stress related chemicals is significantly reduced. That includes corticotropin releasing hormone, the molecule that contributes to anxiety and the initial drop in serotonin, as well as cortisol, which at high levels can impair memory and cause fat to be unhealthfully deposited in your midsection. The question asked by scientists was why? Was it because sucrose tastes good and counters the negative feelings associated with stress, or was it because the extra sugar was somehow fueling parts of the brain capable of turning off the stress response? To answer that question, the investigators infused the solution directly into the rat's stomach. It didn't work. To be effective, the taste buds had to be stimulated. Next, the scientists substituted water flavored with Saccharine, an artificial sweetener. It was just as effective as the sucrose. The conclusion was that just exposure to the taste of something sweet was enough to attenuate the stress response. Thus, it was the hedonic, not metabolic properties of the solution that exerted the effect.

No wonder nurses let infants taste something sweet prior to an invasive procedure. No one has ever measured the chemistry involved, but it doesn't really need doing. After all, converting a scream to a whimper is pretty convincing evidence that this is an effective strategy in humans as well.

In the laboratory study, not only were the chemicals of stress reduced, but stress-behaviors as well. Providing the sweet water prior to being stressed resulted in more socialization, and exploration, an indication of reduced anxiety. Even more remarkable is the fact that the stress buffering effects lasted for up to 7 days after drinking the water. Further investigation revealed the reduced neuroendocrine, sympathetic, and anxiety behaviors were mediated by reward circuitry in the brain. While the effects were modest, indeed only about a 10 to 20 percent reduction, that would certainly be enough to entice a person experiencing a large amount of stress to turn to sugary desserts as a way to cope with adversity.

Eventually, the brain will associate the reward of reduced stress with the taste of sweet food without your even thinking about it. It will become a conditioned response, and thus basis for a habit that will find you eating whenever you are faced with a stressful event. Once a habit is formed, the responsible brain circuitry will remain. Therefore, if you have a habit of turning to comfort foods in the wake of adversity, the goal should be to replace the trigger of the response with something non-fattening. Just about anything you find pleasurable will work. The tricky part of the task is to find something that's rewarding, but without the consequences of packing on unwanted, extra calories. Thus, alcohol and drugs should be avoided. Alcohol contains 7 calories per gram, which puts it between carbohydrate and fat. Since it's the hedonic or reward property of the food that's effective, simply using artificial sweeteners should work as well. After all, it did in the rat study.

There's another way carbohydrates, which include sugar, can alleviate stress. John is a marathon runner who decided to accept an even greater challenge; Ultra-distance triathlons. In addition to running, he decided to add competitive swimming and bicycling to his repertoire. The race was still two months away, but he was already immersed in an arduous training schedule during which he spent hours in the pool, on his bike, and pounding the pavement in his running shoes. The goal was to begin the day with a 2.4 mile swim, followed by a 112 mile bike ride, and then a 26 mile run. The premier event is the Ironman competition staged in Hawaii.

He worked with a trainer and felt good throughout the weeks of training. Then the big day arrived. He did a lot better than expected despite the fact this was his first attempt. But within a few days after the finish, he came down with an upper respiratory infection. His friends and family were surprised, after all exercise is supposed to augment not only the cardiovascular system, but the infection fighting immune system. Much to his surprise, he learned this was not uncommon, especially amongst highly competitive endurance athletes. The reason is they have the perfect immunologic storm; increased exposure to microbes and decreased immunity.

Throughout training and especially during the event, John was experiencing stress. No, not the type he would have dealt with following the loss of a loved one, or a job. That would be psychogenic stress or the anticipation of trauma. John was experiencing what's known as somatic stress, a result of putting excessive demands on his musculoskeletal and cardiorespiratory systems. Despite the fact he was in control, able to predict when he would be finished, and optimistic he would do well, he nonetheless was placing demands on his body for additional glucose. Then, that sugar had to be pumped throughout his blood stream so it could fuel his muscles. His endocrine system was activated giving rise to the glucose triggering hormone, cortisol. At the same time, his sympathetic nervous system poured out another chemical called epinephrine or adrenaline which increased his heart rate. However, both cortisol and epinephrine can down-regulate the immune system.

At the same time, he was probably in a state of at least mild dehydration. Without adequate fluid, he wasn't able to produce the mucous needed to protect the airways from viral attack. Hence, his immune system was not optimal, while at the same time it was easier for viruses to enter his lungs. It's a very common outcome and the reason many sports doctors encourage endurance athletes like John to limit their events to no more than two per year. However, there are athletes who compete at a far greater frequency than is recommended and they don't get sick. They have discovered that by ingesting a solution containing about 5 percent carbohydrate, they can blunt the stress response, thereby sparing their immune system. It makes perfect sense.

Even in solid form, carbohydrates are more rapidly converted into glucose than either protein or fat. In liquid form, the rise in blood sugar would occur even faster. Remember that the primary purpose of the stress response is to mobilize energy stores to fuel the fight/flight response. That's what cortisol and epinephrine help bring about. But if there is already sufficient glucose circulating in the bloodstream, there would be no need to mobilize these two immunosuppressive hormones to get more. Hence, the immune system would be spared. The liquid carbohydrate accomplishes that. The optimal amount of carbohydrate is to be found in many commercial sports drinks. Manufacturers of running shoes, energy bars, and all the other goods that support the multibillion dollar a year sports industry do not want athletes resting on the couch while recovering from infection. They want them wearing out, or consuming the products so they'll buy more.

I'm explaining this not to encourage you to use these dietary approaches to attenuate your stress. Chances are very good you're already doing them, because stress triggers a craving for carbohydrates. I'm explaining it because when you understand what triggers certain behaviors, it makes it easier to find more healthful ways to achieve the same outcome. Yes, there are many other strategies for modulating stress besides ingesting foods that could add to your waistline.

Causes and Symptoms of Stress

A question posed when the study of stress became a legitimate field of scientific inquiry was, *"Where do the emotions of stress come from?"* Do they originate in the brain or elsewhere in the body? In other words, are you running away because you're afraid, or are you afraid because you are running away? Subsequent research has revealed the answer to be 'YES'. There has to be an initial perception of a potential threat before fear can be experienced. However, once anxiety pathways cause a faster beating heart and the outpouring of stress hormones, these signals eventually travel back to the brain to potentiate the emotion. Therefore, like everything else I've been talking about, there is a stimulus followed by a response with feedback to the brain. In this case, the stimulus is your perception of the event, while your response constitutes the symptoms. From a pragmatic standpoint, this means there are two approaches you can employ when dealing with stress; you can change your perception of events, or you can take steps to attenuate your response. Either strategy will reduce your stress. Here are three options to change your perception.

- Reframe by distracting yourself. Transport yourself in space and time to either a real or imaginary place such as a beach or meadow that will more likely bring about a state of tranquility. This is called guided-imagery and has been found to be highly effective for some people.

- Mindfulness is a process whereby you train yourself to focus on something that is unlikely to evoke an emotion. I've been talking about replacing unhealthy ways of responding to stress with healthy ones. That's what this technique does. You learn to take control so when intrusive thoughts take hold, through practice you can replace them with innocuous images.

- Recall a past stressful event from which you emerged largely unscathed. If it was worse than your current dilemma, even better. It will remind you there are nearly always solutions, and at the same time that things could be worse. As a result, you will experience a sense of optimism, which often is all it takes to begin the recovery process.

Here are three options that will target your symptoms.

- There's a recovery pathway in the brain called the parasympathetic nervous system and you can jumpstart it by taking three deep breathes. This will increase blood levels of oxygen allowing you heart rate to come down. That's the job of the parasympathetic pathways, which will prompt other symptoms such as anxiety to go down as well.

- Moving your head back and forth approximating what you might experience in a rocking chair will increase the blood pressure close to sensors in your neck. When pressure goes up, they bring it down by reducing heart rate. This is another way to activate the brain's recovery pathway. Rocking will spill over and help reduce other symptoms of stress as well.

- Walk briskly for twenty minutes. At the end, you'll experience the release of endorphins. That word is a contraction of endogenous-morphine. The reason this brain chemical was given that name is because on a molecular basis, it's as powerful a pain killer as morphine and helps to induce a feeling of wellbeing.

There are many other stress-management approaches you can employ as well. Chances are there are some you may already be using. It doesn't matter which one you choose. Massage, sitting in a sauna, and being with friends are just a few of the options. What's important is that whatever you do should be equal and the opposite of what is causing your stress. Therefore, if your burnout is due to too much tedium bordering on boredom, then recovery should be in the form of something stimulating. Learn to speak a foreign language, or audition for a part in a community theater production.

On the other hand, if your stress is due to excessive energy expenditure because you are on your feet all day, then listening to relaxing music while sitting in a comfortable chair might be the solution. In addition, there are active forms of stress recovery such as meditation or prayer, and active forms such as stretching and swimming. The key to success is to choose a form of recovery that counters the stress you are experiencing. Remember, stress is a major trigger of excessive eating, especially sugar and fat laden foods. Therefore, anything you do to alleviate stress is going to help you lose weight. One of the ways it causes you to eat more is by reducing the amount and quality of your sleep.

Sleeping Less Makes You Eat More

Sleep deprivation is correlated with weight gain, in part because sleeping less can lead to eating more. It makes sense. Even though you may be exhausted, as you lay in bed, ruminating about everything going wrong with your life, your brain thinks you are active. If you are active, then you probably need food and the appetite centers in the brain will be turned on. Since stress is the reason you can't sleep, the foods you select are likely to be those that can quickly be converted into energy. It's been estimated that not getting enough sleep is correlated with the daily consumption of 20 percent or more additional calories compared with when in a fully rested state. There are other symptoms of sleep deprivation as well. These include sadness, irritability, difficulty making decisions, as well as a sense of hopelessness and helplessness. In other words, the symptoms of depression, which can independently lead to changes in eating habits. Therefore, taking steps to get the sleep you need should be a part of your weight loss protocol. These are some things you can do to help achieve a good night's sleep.

Begin by restricting what you do in the bedroom. Earlier, I spoke about conditioning in the context of eating. It turns out that sleep is one of the easiest behaviors to condition. Laboratory animals can be trained to fall asleep at the drop of a pin. You may not realize it but there are probably a large number of conditioned cues that you rely upon to fall asleep. Time of day is an obvious one, but watching the late news or reading a book might be others. They have become such ingrained parts of your routine you do them automatically. The same is true of objects in the bedroom. The bedside lamp, pictures on the wall along with the pillows help to trigger the sleep cycle. Suppose that instead of falling asleep, when your head hits the pillow you find yourself wide awake worrying about all the problems at work. All those cues that normally trigger sleep will eventually become paired with worrying. Even though you are exhausted, the nightly ritual of watching the news, turning on the bedroom light, and taking in your surroundings will turn on the worry cycle. When your head hits the pillow, you'll pick up where you left off the night before. That's why it's necessary to get out of bed as soon as you realize the worrying is a barrier to sleep.

Worrying is actually good for you. It's a form of higher processing whereby you compare what is happening in the present, with circumstances that have occurred in the past, then attempt to predict what the future outcome is likely to be. It's only when the worrying interferes with what you need to get done (such as falling sleep) that it becomes a problem. Get out of bed to avoid associating sleep cues with worrying. Then go to a part of the house to get the worrying out of your system. It will still interfere with your sleep, but at least you're doing it on your terms, and you'll avoid forming an association with the bedroom. Even better, set aside about 20 minutes each day to worry. Do it on your terms. Select a time of day when it's least likely to interfere with your productivity or pleasure. But don't sit in your favorite chair or else it will become paired with the worry cycle. 20 to 30 minutes is about right. Less than 20 minutes is probably insufficient time to make progress to arriving at a solution, while more than 30 minutes will probably cut into the time required to complete other important tasks.

Eat carbohydrates to fall asleep faster. The rise in insulin that follows a carbohydrate rich meal facilitates the transport of tryptophan across the blood brain barrier. Once in the brain, this amino acid can be converted into serotonin, the neurotransmitter that helps lull you to sleep. It's why you often feel sleepy after eating more lasagna or spaghetti than you perhaps should have. Avoid that type of food at lunch when you need to concentrate in the afternoon, but by all means select that item for dinner when you anticipate a sleepless night. As always, do so in moderation.

Lower Your Body Temperature

Deep in your brain there's a thermostat, which determines what your temperature should be. When you're sick, the thermostat is turned up so you can experience a disease fighting fever. But when you sleep, the thermostat is turned down so your temperature drops. It's that drop in temperature that triggers the onset of sleep. You can assist your body in achieving this optimal state by keeping the bedroom on the cool side. High 60s to about 70 degrees appears optimal for most people. Too hot or too cold and the body has to work extra hard to get your temperature to the set-point. That will either keep you awake or cause you to awaken in the middle of the night.

You can actually induce a drop in body temperature with very little effort by taking a hot bath or shower just before going to bed. Initially, the heat will cause your body temperature to rise. If you've ever been in a sauna, you know that perspiring is a common reaction to the heat. Your body is using the sweating mechanism to prevent your body temperature from exceeding 98 degrees. When you immerse your body in warm water, your brain will activate physiological processes to keep your body at the set-point. When you turn the shower off, or step from the hot-tub, the cooling mechanisms will remain activated for a while, resulting in a lowering of your temperature. If the transition from heat to room temperature occurs abruptly, the body often overcompensates resulting in your temperature dropping even lower than intended. That's when you feel sleepy. People often take a hot bath before going to bed in order to relax. It may well do that, but the drop in temperature is the more powerful inducer of sleep. Take advantage of it, especially on nights when you have a lot on your mind and are likely to toss and turn.

There are other things you can do as well, although 'shouldn't do' is more accurate. Many people recognize that drinking coffee after a certain time keeps them from falling asleep. That's because caffeine activates some of the same brain mechanisms that provide energy to mobilize the fight/flight response. The energy might be welcome in the morning when you need to jumpstart the day. However, the anxious feeling excess caffeine may induce could be a barrier to restful sleep. Coffee is not the only source of caffeine. Coffee sets the upper bar with about 200-300 mg per 16 fl oz., however, the same amount of brewed tea comes in at a close second at 100-250. Other chemicals found in tea help to offset the stimulatory effects, but it's still high. 12 oz. of Mountain dew, Dr. Pepper, and Pepsi are 54, 43, and 38 mg respectively while a 1.45 oz. Hershey's dark chocolate bar comes in at 30 mg. There's nothing wrong with consuming caffeinated beverages. However, if you are having difficulty falling asleep at night, it might be worth taking steps to reduce your caffeine intake, especially close to bedtime.

It's not uncommon for those experiencing a great deal of stress to drown their sorrows with a glass of wine or some other form of alcohol. They find it helps them to relax and fall asleep. While that may be true for some people, the alcohol could become a conditioned stimulus, so after a period of time, you cannot sleep without having a nip. In addition, while alcohol may decrease the latency to fall asleep, it may impair the quality of that sleep. Research has found alcohol will increase the time spent in delta or slow wave sleep during the first half of the sleep cycle, and then disrupt it during the second half. Therefore, alcohol should not be used a sleep aid. The ultimate goal is to avoid sleep deprivation, and the increased eating, which lack of sleep can cause.

Excess Food

The obesogenic environment is characterized by other factors as well, including federal legislation regulating agriculture dating back to the 1970's. Dr. Carson Chow is an MIT educated mathematician and physicist who developed a mathematical model to explain the obesity epidemic in the United States. His model is based in part upon a comparison of the food environment when farmers were subsidized to grow less food, with the post-legislative period when they were granted financial incentives to grow more. The major difference? Food became more abundant and cheaper. By 2005, the average American was consuming an additional 1000K calories per day, and the rate of obesity had climbed from 20 to 30 percent. Not only that, but restaurants, including the fast food industry, thrived by selling super-sized meals at bargain prices. Eating out was a rare treat in the 1950's. It was a ritual reserved to celebrate special occasions. When federal legislation increased the supply of food, prices plummeted and eating out became routine with restaurants available at just about any price-point. Ray Kroc had earlier revolutionized the distribution of food by transforming a small family owned restaurant in California called McDonald's into a world-wide chain of franchised restaurants. Others followed suit with the result that a person now has the ability to consume more calories in a single meal than they need for an entire day. Not only that, but times have changed, so the same meal we consume may be far more energy dense than what our parents consumed. For example, twenty years ago, the average size of a bagel was three inches and it packed about 140 calories. The average size of today's bagel has doubled to 6 inches and packs about 350 calories. And that's before it's smeared with cream cheese, which today's bagel will require twice as much of due to the greater size. Chances are, 20 years ago when a person indulged themselves, they had an 8-ounce cup of coffee with a small amount of whole milk and some sugar for a total of 45 calories. Today, the equivalent would more likely be a 16-ounce coffee mocha packing 350 calories. Grab a Double Whopper with a large order of fries and even without a soda, you've added another 1400 calories. Of course not all people consume those foods on a daily basis. My point is, the environment we live in makes it very easy to do so. These types of foods are often as close as the next intersection. Furthermore, you don't even have to step out of your car if you use the drive-thru window. Dr. Chow has used mathematical models of human metabolism and physiology to postulate the push hypothesis to explain the rise in obesity: "Dramatic increases in production, availability, and marketing of cheap, readily available food over the past few decades has led to increased food consumption and obesity along with increased food waste". But that's just the mathematical part.

It wasn't just the changes in agriculture and the distribution of food that occurred during the late 60's and 1970's. The civil rights movement was gaining momentum and in order to facilitate the desegregation of public schools, busing students to distant academic centers became commonplace in many school districts. While no longer used for desegregation purposes, riding in a bus to school has replaced walking or bicycling for many children. Thus, the ritual of beginning and ending each day with exercise is no longer a part of growing up. Other factors such as the elimination of recess and mandatory physical education classes in many school districts have each contributed to the rising rate of childhood obesity. By the way, many habits are formed during childhood. When they become adults, those children will find it exceedingly difficult to replace the firmly engrained familiar eating and exercise habits with new and healthier ones.

Let's revisit for a moment the ramifications of stress and how it factors into the obesity equation. When the going gets tough, we turn to the familiar. We seek out friends and family, and often return to places we know well. Why? The more familiar a person or place is, the more we are able to predict what is likely to happen. That is critical. You see the inability to predict can trigger the one emotion, which more than any other can hold us back in our professional as well as personal endeavors. That emotion is fear. Under duress, we turn to the familiar to reduce both fear and its close cousin, anxiety. That means, you'll be more likely to head to your favorite fast food restaurant when the pressure builds. Let's consider this scenario.

When he was a preschooler, Billy's parents took him to the local McDonald's for special occasions. It was his favorite place because while mom and dad waited in line, he could play in the bouncy ball cage near the entrance. When it was time to sit down, the first thing he did was rip open the box to see what toy was packaged with the Happy Meal. In a very subtle way, Billy was learning to associate McDonald's with pleasure in much the same way Pavlov's dogs learned to salivate upon hearing a bell after the ringing had been paired with the sight and smell of meat. Fast forward a dozen years when Billy and his friends are cramming for their college entrance exams. It's late and they're hungry. They don't want to take too much time from their studies, so off they go to the local McDonald's. Without realizing it, they gravitate to a place they've associated with pleasure since early childhood. What better way to temporarily counter the fear of failure they are all anticipating. Let's fast forward again, about 30 years when Billy finds out he's just lost his job. It's a different stressor, but same response that has him pulling into the local fast food restaurant while driving to his next job interview.

It's important to realize that more and more fast food restaurants are offering healthy choices to their customers. But these are not the choices a stressed out customer is likely to make. It's not McDonald's or any other fast food restaurant that's to blame. It's simply a part of the environment that makes it easy for a person to make unhealthy choices driven primarily by stress related events taking place in the brain. There's one more thing. No matter where you pull in, the burger at one fast food restaurant will taste identical to the one purchased from a restaurant part of the same chain a thousand miles away in another city. The reason is because the flavor does not originate from the burger. That's blasted out when the meat is subjected to ultra-hot steam to destroy harmful microbes. The flavor comes from added chemicals that fool the customer's taste buds into perceiving the flavor of a charbroiled burger. Consequently, the flavor can be preserved over both time and space. That makes it familiar and provides yet another explanation as to why we turn to those types food during times of duress. Your brain is providing the motivation, past experience is providing the pleasure, and familiarity is lessening the fear. They are called comfort foods for a very good reason!

Internal Environment

t's not just the environment we live in that impacts our health; the genetic inspired environment within is at least equally important. I'm sure you know someone who can eat all they want without adding an ounce of extra fat to their body. This part of the program will delve into the many reasons why some people have an easier time with weight management than do others. I'll begin with genetics.

Genetics

Research with identical twins has revealed that when young men are overfed by the same number of additional calories, there is variability in the number of pounds gained. While each twin added about the same amount as his brother, the range between sets of twins was from about 10 to 30 pounds. Scientists interpret this to mean that genetic factors enable some people to increase their basal metabolic rate when they overeat, which is consistent with the set-point hypothesis. It predicts that the body wants to maintain a certain weight and regardless of the diet you are on, will struggle to get back to it. Therefore, it should be as difficult to go above it as below. That is what was found in the twins study. Just as some people have a difficult time establishing a lower body weight set-point, others have a challenge getting to a higher one.

Genes predict probability, not causality. There has to be something that activates or de-activates a particular gene. Such variables are referred to as epigenetic factors and can range from certain types of food to stress. No wonder there is little consensus on the best way to manage body weight, especially those strategies proposed by entrepreneurs wishing to capitalize on the obesity epidemic by selling diet pills and formulas based upon making drastic changes in the proportion of various nutrients. It seems the debate between those claiming to have a better approach have come to rival those that characterize some political campaigns.

The only way to manage weight is to be aware of calories in and calories out. It's that simple. If you want to lose weight, you have to use more calories than you take in. Gaining weight requires consuming more than you burn, and if you want to remain at your current body weight, then you need to be in calorie balance. This book is not about what to do, rather, why CAN'T I and/or why WON'T I? Let's continue with the discussion of why some people have a greater challenge than others when setting about to manage their body weight in a healthful way. Only with this understanding can you customize an approach best suited for your circumstances.

There is evidence there are more than 120 genes associated with obesity. One in particular that has received a large amount of attention is called the fat mass and obesity-associated or FTO gene. About 40-65 percent of the US population possesses at least one copy of this gene, which stimulates appetite and decreases satiety.

Therefore, people with this gene tend to eat more and are less sensitive to feeling full. No wonder they weigh more than people lacking the FTO gene. However, as I mentioned earlier, having a particular gene only increases the probability of experiencing a particular outcome. It is not a guarantee. In the case of those possessing the FTO gene, physical exercise was found to decrease their obesity risk by 27 percent.

When I was asked to design a wellness program for a large hospital, I began by asking the future participants why they weren't already taking steps to get healthy. "Being overweight runs in my family" was a very common answer. It very well may have been true, in which case it probably had become an excuse to ignore taking steps to modify the genetic factors. A study revealed that when people learned they had a gene predisposing them to obesity, within 6 months they were consuming more fat and had reduced their amount of physical activity. It's as though they decided, what's the point? My genes will find a way to pack the fat away so why should I waste my time trying to stop the inevitable. They might be right, but unfortunately, that attitude may well predispose future generations to the same outcome. Here's the reason why.

Epigenetics

Agouti mice are normally born with a yellow tinge to their fur and soon develop into obese adults prone to cancer and diabetes. When bred, these traits are passed on to their offspring. Clearly, a gene is responsible. But recall that genes have to be activated or deactivated to have the predicted outcome. Scientists found that by simply changing the mother's diet just before conception, they could turn the obesity gene off. This simple dietary manipulation resulted in offspring with normal coloring and body weight. Genes are a set of instructions for a specific protein. By feeding the mothers-to-be a diet containing a nutrient capable of turning the agouti gene off, the proteins normally produced in response to that gene were absent. Hence, no yellow fur, no obesity, no diabetes and no cancer. Those studies conducted at Duke University in 2003 ushered in a new field of study called nutrigenomics. It's the study of how genes are impacted by the environment and nutrition.

That's all well and good if you're concerned about the health of your pet mouse. What about humans? Is there evidence our genes are likewise influenced by simply changing the diet? Controlled studies would be difficult to conduct, however, population studies suggest the answer is 'yes'. For example, it may help explain why some people on the identical diet and engaging in the same amount of exercise will lose variable amounts of body weight, while others may even gain weight. In other words, they had the same intake and expenditure of calories, yet vastly different outcomes.

Studies of those consuming moderate amounts of red wine as part of the plant based Mediterranean Diet have shown they have a reduced incidence of cardiovascular disease. But only if they possess a particular set of genes. Without those genes, alcohol has no protective effect upon the heart. Similarly, not all ethnic groups who consume a high-fat Western diet experience the same susceptibility to heart disease. That might well be due to genetic differences, as well as the observation that women who consume a surplus of food during certain stages of pregnancy are more likely to give birth to offspring who later develop type 2 diabetes. It's too early to create designer recipes capable of reliably eradicating disease, and it may be a while before that day arrives. After all, the human genome is comprised of approximately 25,000 genes having millions of variations. Add gender, age, metabolic factors, as well as a host of non-food related environmental factors, and it becomes clear that it will be years before we can make that sometimes quantum leap from the laboratory to the human clinic. But while it may be premature to start manipulating genes, there are things you can do to influence the biological events dictated by genes, especially those pertaining to metabolism.

Metabolism

Genes dictate the types of proteins we produce and without question influence every process that transpires in the human body, including those linked with body weight. Some of those influences may be working through biological events also linked directly or indirectly with body weight. I'll begin by reviewing the metabolic events.

Your thyroid is the endocrine gland that is most influential in regulating metabolism. People producing low amounts of thyroid hormone are likely to have reduced metabolism, which will slow the burning of extra calories. Predictably, people with low metabolism and not just secondary to thyroid problems, are at greater risk of gaining weight. Compared with those with normal or high metabolism, they will also have a more difficult time losing weight. Other factors besides the thyroid can also influence metabolism.

People with a larger amount of lean tissue, or muscle, will have a greater basal metabolic rate compared with those having more adipose or fat tissue. That is something you can influence through weight bearing exercise. The more muscle or lean tissue you have, the more calories you will burn even when engaged in sedentary behavior. Of course it goes without saying that physical activity will speed metabolism, so it's no surprise that those who are active will be less likely to experience weight gain. Conversely, inactivity is correlated with increased weight gain.

Sympathetic Nervous System

Another factor that will increase energy expenditure is the sympathetic nervous system. The chemicals produced when this system is activated, are responsible for many of the symptoms normally associated with stress, such as, increased heart rate, increased respiration rate, and dry mouth. It works with the cortisol producing endocrine pathway to both increase available energy, as well as to propel it quickly to the cells that may need it, hence, the increase in heart rate and blood pressure. Some people have less sympathetic tone or activity than others, which will predispose them to weight gain.

Fat Oxidation

Ultimately, it is fat tissue that a person wants to lose. Not muscle, which as noted can assist with weight management by increasing the basal metabolic rate. Actually, carbohydrate is the most efficient nutrient to burn because of its comparatively faster rate of conversion into blood sugar. However, some people are more predisposed to burn carbohydrate thereby sparing their fat stores. They have what is called a low fat oxidation rate. There is a way to speed the burning of fat. Athletes exercise to improve their strength and agility; others find exercise relaxing, while some people work out to lose weight. Different forms of exercise are optimal depending upon your objective. Aerobic workouts will benefit sprinters and those wishing to increase their endurance, while weight training will benefit those seeking to increase their strength. Later, I'll explain why exercise for a long time at moderate intensity is best for burning fat.

Steps to Increase Metabolism

In addition to reducing the intake of calories, burning them faster is another option if you want to lose weight. But be careful because sometimes the claims are not supported by scientific data. In some instances, the studies haven't been conducted, and in others, the studies don't always support the marketing claims. The following foods have been claimed to increase metabolism. In a few instances, they may help you shed a few pounds somewhat.

- Caffeine has been shown to increase overall metabolism and fat oxidation in a dose dependent manner, which means the more you ingest the higher your metabolism will go. Caffeine also synergizes with the green tea ingredient, catechin, which independently increases metabolism. However, the impact on weight loss is minimal and after ingesting these ingredients over time, the effects are reduced.

- Carnitine is a nutrient that helps transport fatty acids across the mitochondria membrane, which is where food is ultimately converted into energy. Because of this well documented effect, carnitine has been marketed as a weight loss strategy. However, there is no scientific evidence to support this claim.

- Capsaicin is a spice found in hot peppers. For each teaspoon added to a meal, it has been found to increase energy expenditure by up to 1.5 calories. The same has been found true of milder sweet peppers, which happen to be a good source of vitamin C, beta-carotene and a host of beneficial phytochemicals.

- Cold water has to be brought up to body temperature after entering the stomach. This will increase metabolism as part of water induced thermogenesis. Of course anytime heat is generated, calories are being burned. Studies have shown that drinking 500 ml of room temperature water will increase energy expenditure by 30 percent over a time period of about forty minutes. Theoretically, drinking 12 ounces of cold water could burn an additional 22 calories per day, which translates into about 2 pounds of weight loss per year. It's not a lot, but losing two pounds is much better than gaining that amount.

- Fish oil was found in some initial studies to increase lean body mass and thereby increase metabolic rate. In fact, some people still cling to the belief it may help. However, subsequent studies have been unable to confirm this finding. There are numerous other benefits associated with fish oil, so why not try it even though weight loss has not been proven.

- Grapefruit diets have been in vogue off and on for years. Studies have shown that eating half a

grapefruit at each meal will result in the loss of
about 3.5 pounds within 12 weeks. What is not
clear is why. Some have suggested it is due to
an appetite suppressing chemical, while others
think it may have more to do with the appetite
suppressing effects of the acidic taste or extra
bulk.

- Of all the strategies to increase metabolism and
thereby burn fat calories, exercise is by far the
best.

Another approach is to take advantage of the appetite
suppressing effects of protein. This macronutrient has
been found to increase metabolism, and to also activate
satiety centers in the brain. Consequently, a person will
stop eating sooner and wait longer before eating again.
In addition, the amino acids comprising protein are
needed to build muscle. As I noted earlier, muscle burns
calories at a faster rate than fat cells so the mere presence
of lean body mass will burn additional calories.

The appetite suppressing effects of protein is something that impacted me in a way I was neither expecting nor seeking. I belong to an organization called
WaterTribe, which hosts extreme adventure races using
small, human powered boats. In 2006 I completed the
inaugural 1240-mile Ultimate Challenge. It was a circumnavigation of Florida, which took almost a month to
complete in an 18 foot decked canoe. There was ample
space to carry supplies, so I always had food to eat and
snack on. My inventory happened to include a large sup-

ply of protein bars given to me by a sponsor. When I completed the race, I had lost over 20 pounds. I couldn't understand why since I had plenty of food so was able to eat whenever I wanted. However, because the extra protein made me feel full when I really needed more calories, I was in negative calorie balance. In other words, the all-day physical exertion that stretched over a month was burning more calories that I was taking in. When I got home clothes didn't fit and I had no extra energy for almost a month. That's how long it took me to gain back the weight I had lost. For me, it was not desired, however, if your goal is to lose weight, consider the protein option. Be careful. Protein is comprised of amino acids, which contains nitrogen. If not cleared quickly from the body, it will be converted into ammonia and then urea before being flushed through the kidneys. Damage can occur if a sufficient amount of water is not consumed while digesting a large amount of protein.

I've given you a lot of information regarding how the body works in the context of food intake and metabolism. I'll come back later to this discussion along with more things you can with this understanding. At this time, I want to focus on the most important part of a weight management program; motivation to proceed with a strategy and then stay with it.

Am I Ready to Lose Weight?

t's one thing to say you are, it's quite another matter to put the words into action. Start by reviewing your history so you can identify potential obstacles. Have you ever tried to lose weight before, and if so how long were you able to adhere to the protocol? If the time was a certain number of days or weeks, then you probably weren't ready at the outset. You just thought you were. If you stuck with it for several months, then chances are something happened to disrupt your new routine. Reflect back upon the circumstances that existed. Were you under a lot of stress? Did you stop around the time of a major family event such as a wedding where a large meal is typically served? Or perhaps the stumbling block was a major holiday, many of which are celebrated with the consumption of food. If that's what derailed your plans, chances are you viewed yourself as a failure and decided to not risk experiencing that feeling again.

Consider this strategy. Measure your success not on a daily basis, but on a weekly or even biweekly basis. Remember, success is making progress toward a worthwhile goal. It's up to you, but I would include a daily, weekly, and monthly goal. A weekly goal is especially important because it will allow enough days to counter the one or two days when you let your guard down. Then, give yourself a reward for meeting your goal. It might be an evening at the movies, going to your favorite place such as a beach or park, or attending a concert or sporting event. Here's an example of what I'm referring to:

Don't make your weekly goal all or nothing. If you weren't able to stay with your plan before, then chances are you may stumble again. But you don't have to feel like a failure when that happens. Perhaps you didn't lose any weight; however, a week of not gaining weight is good, so give yourself partial credit, perhaps one point. Actually losing weight earns more, for example one point for each pound lost. So if you lost two pounds at the end of a particular week, you get one point for not gaining weight, plus two more for the pounds lost. Give yourself a score of three for the week. The next week may find you having lost three pounds, which means it was a four-point success (one for not gaining, and three for each pound). Whoops. The next week finds you with an extra pound on the scale's dial. That will net you minus points corresponding to the number of pounds you gained. Once you complete a month, start keeping a monthly score as well. That way, even though one of the weeks might have included Thanksgiving Day, your monthly score will probably still be in the success column despite that one off-week. By doing it this way, you still chalk up a success.

Remember, your goal is to lose weight, but your measure of success is simply making progress toward that goal. Shedding pounds is one metric of success, but not necessarily the most reliable one. As you consume fewer calories than you are using, you'll burn some stored fat to make up the difference. However, as you increase the time you exercise, you'll accumulate more muscle, which happens to weigh more than fat. In other words, you may not see any progress on the scale if they cancel each other. Indeed, you may even reach a point where you start gaining a bit. Nonetheless, you may still be making progress toward your goal. Here's how you find out.

There are easy to use devices that measure the percentage of fat. They're not as accurate as underwater weighing and other more sophisticated techniques, but will work fine for your purposes. They come configured as a set of scales you'd stand on to weigh yourself or a device you hold in your hand to measure electrical impedance. Since the flow of electrical current varies depending upon whether it's passing through water attracting muscle versus water aversive fat, it can be interpreted as an approximation of your total body fat. It doesn't have to be accurate, just consistent. What you are interested in is the change during the process of cutting back on calories and adding exercise to your daily routine.

Energy

Most people could care less about losing weight. Instead, they want the things that excess body fat interferes with. For example, a trim figure, more energy, or the ability to pursue more physical activities. Think of a way to quantify what you are seeking and then monitor your progress.

For the sake of illustration, let's pick having more energy as an objective. Many of the people who attend my lectures complain of fatigue. A trip to the grocery store leaves them feeling tired, and despite getting 8 to 10 hours of uninterrupted sleep, they awaken feeling exhausted. No, they don't have Chronic Fatigue Syndrome, the poorly understood condition characterized by post-exertion-fatigue and a host of other major and minor criteria. Nor is the fatigue experienced by many people secondary to cancer or a metabolic disorder. The number one cause of generalized fatigue is sedentary behavior. I realize it sounds counter-intuitive; after all, most people get tired following exercise, not energized. The fact is a short episode of exercise will energize you better than a cup of the strongest coffee you may drink. While working out, you are placing demands on your body for more glucose, which must be rushed to the muscle cells that need it. Of course oxygen is required to convert the glucose into usable energy. Well, the same glucose pool that energizes muscles provides what the brain needs to be in the ideal performance state. Once you begin a regular exercise program, you will find you have more overall energy than you did prior to starting. See for yourself. Using a scale of one to ten, keep track of how much energy you have each morning. One is equivalent to being in a coma and ten has you feeling up to completing a triathlon. Do it again in the early afternoon and a third time in the evening. As you make gains in getting healthier, increased energy will be a part of your reward. Keep track of it and as your energy level increases, take credit for having made it happen. Use the same approach to monitor anything that you might want to change as part of your quest for optimal health. Don't limit your measure of success to just body weight.

Choosing a Strategy That's Right for You

Many dietary strategies have been marketed to those seeking to lose weight. Most assuredly, new ones are on the horizon. It is beyond the scope of this book to describe them all. Instead, I'll point out some red flags to look for before you decide, as well as a general approach that will help you achieve a state of optimal body weight with whichever approach you decide to embrace. Be forewarned that marketers are primarily responsible to their shareholders, not the end user of their product. Yes, they want people to succeed and entice their friends to sign on, but ultimately the motive for making the approach or product available is profit. The following are red-flags:

- The claim that the strategy is based a new discovery should be taken as a warning. If it really is new, then it is doubtful that well-controlled research has been carried out to verify the claims. If it isn't, then you're dealing with a company engaging in deception. Either way, avoid the approach.

- Any program that claims you can lose weight without exercising is bogus. Losing weight requires burning more calories than you are taking in. Without exercising, you'd have to restrict your calorie intake so much; it would likely impact the intake of vitamins and minerals thereby leaving you prone to undernutrition. There are essential fatty acids and amino acids that can be obtained only through the ingestion of food. That means some calories are inevitable if you want to remain healthy. The key is to grab the micronutrients, then burn the calories that accompanied them.

- Conveying the impression that a product has limited availability is a key sales strategy that works. It's the principal of the Black Friday post-Thanksgiving sales which will find people standing for hours in long lines in order to buy one of the three available items at that price. The same is done in the diet industry, except in a more subtle way. To achieve success, you must purchase a rare ingredient made available only by the company selling the product. In addition, they might point out it grows on an inaccessible island in the South Pacific, causing an unsuspecting customer to want it even more.

- The more rigid a diet is, the less healthy it's likely to be. That's because you need variety as reflected in lots of colors and shapes on your plate. That generally means you're getting an assortment and correct balance of vitamins, minerals and phytochemicals to keep the body's metabolic machinery running smoothly. Any diet that restricts the intake of certain vegetables or fruits, or an entire category of macronutrient, such as fat, protein, or carbohydrate could be risky. Yes, there are some medical conditions that necessitate leaving certain foods off your plate. Those suffering from celiac disease should avoid gluten, and people with food allergies should take great pains to avoid eating the source of the allergen. But not the person who is simply trying to lose a few pounds.

- If, in addition to a dietary plan, you are instructed to take supplements to assure the success of the program, be wary. A well balanced diet will provide you with all the ingredients you need.

You cannot dispute data. Numbers are numbers and cannot be ignored. However, you can and you always should dispute the interpretation of data. That includes claims about any particular diet. Many people begin a high carbohydrate diet and quickly start losing pounds. Others experience the same outcome after following a high protein, or high fat diet. Their reduced body weight represents the indisputable data. Why they lost the weight is subject to interpretation. It could be the dietary regimen, or it could be that a person who goes to the trouble of carefully selecting the foods they eat may be doing other things as well. For example, they might be limiting their portion size or exercising more in order to achieve a state of negative calorie balance. Remember, you must have that in order to lose weight. By the way, studies have shown that most any diet a person goes on will enable them to lose weight, but only if they reduce calorie intake and incorporate exercise into their lifestyle. However, it is true that some diets may make it easier for a person to do that. Let's take a careful look at the three main types of diet that have been embraced by some Americans.

Moderate Fat and Protein with High Carbohydrates

Weight Watchers and Jenny Craig diets typically follow the ratio of high carbohydrates recommending that 55 to 60 percent of the total calorie intake be in that form. 20 to 30 percent of the calories should be in the form of fat and the remaining 15 to 20 percent should be in the form of protein. The diet also calls for a deficit of approximately 500 to 1000 calories per day. This can best be accomplished by keeping the calorie intake at no more than 1200 per day for women and no more than 1400 calories for men. Of course combining the reduced caloric intake with increased exercise will speed up the loss of weight, although the recommended goal is no more than 1 to 2 pounds per week. For years, this approach has been the gold standard since many people who lose weight this way also experience healthier levels of blood triglycerides and LDL cholesterol. However, long term follow-up reveals that while there might be initial successes, over an extended time the weight loss is not sustained at a statistically significant level.

High Fat and Protein with Low Carbohydrates

The Atkins Diet Revolution and Sugar Busters are diets that are just the opposite of the Jenny Craig and Weight Watchers recommendation. Instead of carbohydrates, it is recommended that 55 to 65 percent of the daily caloric intake be in the form of fat, with most of the rest as protein. The objective is to reduce appetite by causing ketosis. This happens when there is insufficient carbohydrate in the diet to support the full processing of fat in the cells' energy producing pathway resulting in the buildup of ketone bodies. Research of people subscribing to this strategy is limited, although what has been published reveals people who take this approach do lose weight during at the least the first year in a manner similar to those adopting the opposite strategy. It's also noteworthy that a lot of water is required to flush protein factors out of the body. Many people on high protein diets lose a very large amount of weight during the first week; however, much of it is due to the loss of fluid. Protein also has a longer lasting satiety effect enabling a person to go longer without feeling hungry after consuming a high protein meal. The important question is whether the weight loss reported by those on these types of diet is sustainable. The answer will have to await the completion of long-term studies.

Low Fat, Moderate Protein, and High Carbohydrates

There are different forms of this approach, which was originally designed to decrease the incident of heart disease. Some prescribe a low amount of fat comprising only 11 to 19 percent of the total daily caloric intake. A very low fat-version calls for less than 10 percent fat in the diet. The Ornish Program for Reversing Heart Disease is a vegetarian diet, while the New Pritikin Program allows lean meat, but not to exceed 3.5 ounces per day. Both also recommend regular exercise. While not designed for weight loss, people who adhere to the recommendations of a low or very low fat diet do lose weight. However, supplementation with fat soluble vitamins and some minerals is often necessary since absorption of these nutrients requires adequate fat in the diet. These low fat diets should not be followed by those with diabetes or with malabsorption illnesses.

It seems that exceptions are always the rule in biology and medicine. Thus, for every person who loses weight on a popular diet, another will meet with failure. It may have less to do with motivation than the myriad of factors that have a place in the weight-loss equation. Earlier, I described the role of genetics, epigenetics, metabolic rate as well as other weight-modulatory factors. Therefore, one size never has nor will it ever fit all. If a dietary approach makes sense, then by all means try it. However, if you have any type of medical problem, consult with a Registered Dietician or a health care provider with in-depth nutrition training and experience with the illness of concern. In my opinion, it doesn't matter which diet you subscribe to as long as you do the following:

- Avoid making abrupt changes in caloric intake. You'll be more likely to succeed when taking gradual steps to lose weight.
- Incorporate a regular regimen of exercise into your daily routine. Make it a habit and do it even when you may not want to bother.
- Be cognizant of your eating behavior and then take steps to modify it in order to achieve your desired body weight goal.

Of these, perhaps the most important one is to avoid an abrupt change. You don't want to lose weight too quickly. If you've been carrying excess weight for a long time, your brain has adjusted to the status quo and will resist change. By losing weight gradually, the appetite centers will be less likely to strongly resist your efforts.

The television personality, Oprah Winfrey, went on a well-publicized diet during the course of which she lost a significant amount of weight. However, she eventually regained it as part of what is referred to as the yoyo effect. This phenomenon can be explained by the Set-Point hypothesis, which is predicated upon the belief that the body is engineered to maintain body weight within a very narrow range based upon the person's current weight, not necessarily their healthy weight. Over a period of time, the current weight becomes the set-point regardless of whether it's too much. If a person deviates, changes occur to get the person's weight back to the set point, especially if the weight loss is abrupt. Indeed, a person can experience large variations in daily food intake without a significant change in body weight so long as the average consumption of calories over a year remains about the same. That's because it can take as long as three years for the body to shift to a new set-point. Until the shift occurs, the body will be working through slower metabolism to get your weight back to where it had previously been. When basal metabolic rate slows, less energy is being expended making it more difficult to lose those extra pounds.

Three years is a long time to depend upon willpower to resist the physiology that's lobbying the brain to get you to eat more to maintain the starting set-point. Eventually, it may happen. Research shows that if a person eats 100 fewer calories per day, after three years they will have lost about 10 pounds and once the body accepts the new weight as the norm, it will be easier to maintain it.

Want What You Need

There are two equally important functions of food; the capacity to provide energy and structural components for the body, and the capacity to provide pleasure. These are also referred to as the metabolic and hedonic properties of food. A person must be motivated to seek out and then consume those foods capable of meeting their needs. The pleasurable aspect of food drives that motivation. When people lose the capacity to detect savory flavors, their motivation to eat declines resulting in weight loss and undernutrition. A decline in taste is often associated with advanced age, which is why the elderly are subject to this condition, as are those being treated for cancer using drugs that erode the sensation of savoriness. Both are sapped of their motivation to eat.

It is so important that the body obtain required nutrients that we have very powerful brain chemistry driving us to not only eat, but to select those foods we might be most in need of, especially during times of duress.

Unfortunately, the brain prioritizes the desire for energy foods, which are not always the ones rich in essential nutrients. It becomes even more problematic when we voluntarily restrict our food intake for the purpose of losing weight. That's because our motivation will usually steer us toward quick sources of energy, which are not always the best for maintaining a state of optimal health. That's why this part of program will focus upon why we should always prioritize the consumption of nutritious foods ahead of those that just deliver calories, which often are the good tasting ones. However, we all have a need for pleasure so completely eliminating the tasty morsels is not a good idea. Instead, let's examine ways you can eat the proverbial cake and lose weight as well.

How much of which foods must you consume on a regular basis to maintain a state of optimal health? The best place to turn is to the U.S. Department of Agriculture, which every 5 years' reviews and updates a document called, Dietary Guidelines for Americans. The goal is to offer people scientifically based recommendations to achieve a state of optimal health. Data are collected from experts in nutrition, as well as through public comment. In addition, the interpretation of the data takes into account the general food preferences, and cultural factors found within the diverse groups residing in the U.S. While all data can and should be subject to close scrutiny and re-interpretation when necessary, the Dietary Guidelines for Americans is the best place to start when designing a healthful diet. The USDA guidelines incorporate two interrelated themes; 1. *Maintaining calorie balance over time to achieve and sustain a healthy weight* and *2. Focus on consuming nutrient-dense foods and beverages.* Furthermore, the guidelines strongly recommend that a person meet their nutrient needs through the consumption of foods whenever possible. The consumption of supplements and fortified foods should be avoided unless a specific deficiency warrants it. This is because of potential toxicity when the body is exposed to excess quantities of certain vitamins and minerals.

Maintain a Healthful Diet

This is what you need to know. There are two general categories of food; those that are energy dense and those that are nutrient dense. Most foods contain both, however, in different proportions. You need both. Energy in the form of calories is essential to keep the body running smoothly. But without nutrients, the energy would not burn efficiently and critical parts of the body, such as the brain and immune system, would fail to function as designed. Nutrients are associated with foods that contain calories. Therefore, you will get some of both whenever you eat. Your goal then is to eat foods that provide the greatest amount of nutrients for the lowest possible number of calories. This is not my recommendation, it's the first of four arrived at by some of the nation's top nutritionists who were responsible for developing the Dietary Guidelines for Americans. There are actually twenty-three, and if you want to read all of them, you can by logging onto www.cnpp.usda.gov.

Here are the three main ones:

1. Balance Calories with Physical Activity to Maintain Weight.
2. Consume more of certain foods and nutrients such as fruits, vegetables, whole grains, fat-free and low fat dairy products, and seafood.
3. Consume fewer foods with sodium (salt), saturated fats, trans fats, cholesterol, added sugars, and refined grains.

Let's explore each of these in depth.

Balance calories with physical activity if you want to lose weight. By reducing calorie dense foods you'll take in less, and by increasing exercise, you'll burn more. What are examples of calorie vs nutrient dense foods? Let's start with a low nutrient breakfast, the type you should avoid. A slice of white toast with one teaspoon of butter, half a cup of whole milk and puffed rice cereal is an example. The white, refined bread is going to send your blood sugar into the red zone, while the butter and whole milk are rich in fat, which packs 9 calories per gram. Try instead this high nutrient equivalent. Replace the white bread with whole wheat toast so you get the nutrients found in the bran and germ of the intact grain. Then, reduce the fat content by pouring the same amount of skim instead of whole milk. By replacing the puffed rice cereal with oatmeal, you'll be getting soluble fiber which has multiple health benefits but without the calories. It's the same basic breakfast, including butter on the toast, but healthier. Do the same at lunchtime. Replace a 3oz ground beef hamburger in a white bun with the same amount of turkey breast nestled between two slices of whole-grain bread. Go ahead and put two teaspoons of Dijon mustard on both, after all you want the flavor, but replace the tablespoon of ketchup with three slices of fresh tomato. Use red leaf instead of iceberg lettuce. You'll get the equivalent flavor plus additional nutrients. Then, replace the chips or fries that typically come with a burger with a cup of baby carrots with broccoli crowns. Finally, dump the soda. It's nothing but sugar water with artificial colors and flavors. You're much better off with water. There is no requirement to suffer with bland food while getting healthy. By making just a few substitutions, you can enjoy most of the same flavors while reducing calories and increasing the nutrients. The general rule is the more color you have on your plate, the better off you'll be.

The guidelines recommend a combination of improved eating and physical activity as a way of achieving healthful body weight. That's because nutrition and exercise constitute two sides of the same coin. Calories are a measure of energy, and they are stored mostly as fat. Therefore, to lose fat, your body must engage in a process that consumes energy or in other words, calories. Of course every breath you take and each beat of your heart uses energy. So does the generation of heat from muscles to maintain your body temperature at 98 degrees. Indeed, a certain number of calories are being burned even while you sleep. However, not enough are burned for the average person to shed months or years worth of extra fat calories that have accumulated in unsightly places. So how much exercise is required to burn those extra calories? A widely accepted formula is based upon the educated assumption that the average person burns 1.2 Calories per pound of body weight per hour while walking at a 2 MPH pace. That's a leisurely speed most people would maintain while walking across a parking lot. If a person weighs 200 pounds, they'd need to walk for one hour to burn off the estimated 240 calories in a Starbucks Coffee Frappuccino. If they don't and the calories exceed what they need, they'll be stored as more fat. Here's another way of thinking about it.

An often quoted formula is that 3500 extra calories equals about 1 pound of fat, which means you will need to burn 3,500 more calories than you take in to lose 1 pound. At a two and a half mile pace, that's more than 10 hours of walking per pound. There's a problem with this calculation. It isn't a fixed number of calories that you lose. It's a number that changes significantly during the process of losing weight. Mathematical models developed at the National Institute of Diabetes and Digestive and Kidney Diseases have revealed that the same number of additional calories will add more weight to a fat person than to a thin person. There's a time factor as well because the body will eventually adjust to the existing circumstances, including weight. Therefore, as you take in fewer calories to lose weight, your metabolism will drop as part of a delaying tactic to keep you at your body weight at the level your brain has become accustomed to.

Exercise to Burn Fat. There are many forms of exercise ranging from high intensity activities that leave you breathless, to a leisurely walk at a pace that enables you to still carry on a conversation. Which is best depends upon your goal. If your objective is to burn fat, then less is better. Before I explain why, let's review a few facts pertaining to the burning of fat as energy. Triglycerides are the storage form of fat. They are comprised of glycerol with three fatty acids attached. That's where the energy is located and each fatty acid is classified based upon the number of carbons. The more carbons, the more ATP, which is what drives virtually all the biological events in the body. There are several advantages to storing energy as fat. First, fat contains 9 calories per gram, which is far more than the 4 found in carbohydrate and protein. Second, there is unlimited storage for fat making it an abundant source of energy even in very lean people. Even those with only 10 percent body fat will have an ample supply. For example, a lean runner weighing 160 pounds will have 16 pounds of fat, which is more than 50,000 calories of stored energy. Glucose stored as glycogen provides only about 1,000 to 2,000 kcal. However, the glycogen is going to be available on very short notice. Indeed, muscle has its own glycogen, which is reserved for the exclusive use of that tissue. Fat requires a longer amount of time to become energy. That's why fat is primarily used to fuel the systems that never stop, such as the expansion and contraction of the rib cage while we breathe, or the constant beating of the heart. In general, fat will be used during activities of longer duration and lower intensity. As a consequence, doing less is better if you want to burn fat. A long walk over several hours or long-distance cycling is going to tap into fat stores once the glycogen has been used up. That would happen in about 30 minutes during a moderate paced walk of about 3 to 3.5 miles per hour. Taking a day long hike over 5 to 7 hours would result in 65 percent of energy coming from fat and only 35 percent from carbohydrates. In contrast, running a high intensity marathon over 2.5 to 3 hours would have only 20 percent of the calories coming from fat and 65 percent from carbohydrates. That's because the faster burning carbohydrates would be needed to keep up with the greater intensity of running a marathon. Not only do you burn fat during the exercise, you continue to burn calories for a long time after you stop. You still need to perform other forms of exercise to achieve optimal health. As I noted previously, your strategy should target as many physiological systems as possible.

Here's an example of a healthy routine.

- Spend at least 30 consecutive minutes each day engaging in cardiovascular fitness. Running, brisk walking, cross-country skiing and swimming are examples.
- Do a minimum of 8 to 10 exercises involving the major muscle groups 2 to 3 days per week. For example, push-ups or chin-ups for the arms, shoulders and chest muscles. Crunches and sit-ups are good to firm up the abdominal muscles. Resistance training using weights is another

option. If you want to build endurance, then use lighter weight and more repetitions. For greater strength, use heavier weights with fewer repetitions.

- Do at least 2-4 repetitions of stretching exercises 2 to 4 days per week. Stretch through the full range of motion and hold each stretch for 15 to 30 seconds.

A common question is how you know the intensity is right, especially for building cardiorespiratory health. One option would be to use a heart rate monitor. 50 to 70 percent of your maximum heart rate is defined as moderate intensity while 75 to 85 percent of the maximal is vigorous. By the way, you can determine you approximate maximum heart rate by subtracting your age from 220. It fails to take into account your gender, level of fitness, and medical conditions, as a treadmill test would do. But it will give you an approximation. Another is to use the conversation rule. If you are able to carry on a conversation but would rather not, you are in the moderate range. If the only word you can utter is 'help', you are most likely in the vigorous range. Remember, to burn a maximum amount of fat you need to be in the lower intensity range for several hours.

If you're like many people, you will probably get bored doing one type of exercise for an extended period of time, or keeping track of the number of repetitions. That doesn't have to be the case. A healthy workout that you will stick with should be fun and include variety.

It should also meet both intrinsic and extrinsic needs. The personal satisfaction of having achieved a fitness goal would be an example of an intrinsic factor. However, receiving a reduction in your health insurance cost because you achieved a BMI in the healthful range would be an extrinsic benefit. There's no reason you can't mix things up by combining aerobic with resistance training and stretching. You can also alternate indoor and outdoor activities during the week, and include a variety. For example, there's walking one day, dancing another, with swimming, cycling and gardening in the mix as well. Just don't overdo it. If you are still bored, grab some ear buds and listen to an audio book or music. You'll look forward to the time spent exercising so you can find out 'what happens next'.

Many people buy into the cultural myth that more is better. If you push yourself too hard, the exercise will place demands on your body requiring activation of the stress response in order to adjust. The moment you have to force yourself to summons the motivation to exercise, you should back off. You've most likely crossed into the stress-zone, which is the worst place to be when trying to lose weight.

In the meantime, there are ways to burn extra calories without setting aside specific times to do so.

- Seek out the distant parking space so you get to walk further to the office or shops. Even better, walk to work and take the long route so you can burn more fat calories.
- Always use the stairs instead of the elevator.

- Do sit ups, stretching or walk on a treadmill while watching TV.
- Invite a friend to join you or even better, join a group. When you do things as part of a group, it reinforces your belief that the objective can be achieved. After all, all those people couldn't be wrong, could they? Working out with others also provides a bit more incentive to show up. You're more likely to comply.

Consider going on a physically active vacation. For almost a decade while my children were growing up, our annual family holiday was a 500-mile bicycle ride from the Missouri to the Mississippi River. It was called the Register's Annual Great Bicycle Ride Across Iowa and took a week to complete. It was also a lot of fun, especially since we always did it with friends and neighbors.

Consume more healthful foods. While minimizing the total number of calories consumed, make sure you eat a variety of fruits and vegetables. A general rule of thumb is to make sure you have a variety of color on your plate. Try to include dark green, red, yellow, and orange vegetables as well as legumes such as beans and peas. Make sure while eating carbohydrates, such as breads, pasta and cereals, that they are made from whole grains. Fat is an important nutrient, however, only when consumed in moderation. To avoid an excess, select fat-free or low fat dairy products such as milk, cheese and yogurt. Protein is needed to build muscle, communicate messages from the brain to the rest of the body, along with a host of other critical functions. However, complete protein containing all the amino acids your body needs is often associated with foods that also contain saturated fat, such as beef. Therefore, obtain protein from lean cuts of beef. Remove the fat rich skin from poultry, and try to eat more fish. Eggs, beans and peas, as well as soy products are good sources of protein as well. However, unlike meat, many plants lack certain essential amino acids requiring that you combine vegetables in order to obtain all that you need.

Finally, it's important to include in your diet foods that provide adequate amounts of fiber and those nutrients of concern to nutritionists because some people do not get enough of them. Examples include calcium, potassium and vitamin D. Calcium is critical to maintain healthy bones not to mention the effectiveness of nerve and muscle tissues. Good sources of these nutrients and fiber include fruits, vegetables, legumes, whole grain bread and cereals, and low fat dairy products.

Consume fewer foods with sodium, which is salt, saturated fats, trans fats, cholesterol, added sugars, and refined grains. This is one of the recommendations for the Dietary Guidelines for Americans. The three flavors that impart pleasure via the taste buds are the sweet taste of sugar, the flavor and smooth texture of fat, and salt. Therefore, it is not surprising that many foods are loaded with these ingredients in order to attract customers. All are required, but in moderation. Let's begin with sodium, which is essential for maintaining the required polarity across a cell membrane. This is especially important for neurons, which rely upon electrical conductance to transmit messages, and for muscles to contract. It also draws water into the blood stream to maintain optimal blood pressure. But too much salt will attract an excess of fluid resulting in high blood pressure. While we tend to think of the white substance that pours from a salt shaker as the primary source of dietary salt, the majority of sodium we consume is from prepared meals consumed in restaurants and the processed foods obtained from grocery stores. It is so ubiquitous in our food supply that the average American consumes more than twice what is recommended on a daily basis. In many instances, it's difficult to know exactly how much is present. Food labels will list the amount, however, most people don't keep track. Nor is there any way of knowing what is present in the foods served at a restaurant. Here are some guidelines that might help.

- Choose fresh or just plain frozen vegetables whenever possible. If canned, make sure the label states that no salt has been added.
- Processed meats should be avoided. Cured ham, sausage, bacon as well as most canned meats have a very high salt content.
- Take the time to study the package and read the food label. As you do, realize the average person over the age of two consumes 3400 mg of salt per day. Your goal is to not exceed 2300 mg, and if you can keep your intake to no more than 1500 mg,

that would be best. Seek out those labels that state "low sodium". But be careful not to equate that statement with "no sodium". Many people think that because a food is low in something, they can safely consume more. Even small amounts can start to add up when consumed frequently.

- Add very little, or even better, no additional salt to foods on your plate.
- Be careful of condiments. Ketchup, mustard, pickles, soy sauce, and even olives are additional sources of sodium.

Fat is often demonized in our culture. In excess, it changes a person's appearance in undesirable ways, can lead to obesity and metabolic syndrome, and is able to greatly enhance the likelihood of chronic inflammation. However, you must have it. Fat provides insulation which helps to maintain body temperature, cushions organs, and is necessary to assist with the absorption of the fat soluble vitamins, A, K, and E. The problem is not with fat, but rather the type and amount consumed. Since reducing calories is going to be the prime driver of success no matter which dietary strategy you adopt, reducing fat is going to be imperative. That's because it packs more than twice the calories found in carbohydrates and protein. A gram of fat contains 9 calories compared with just 4 for carbohydrates and protein. In addition, there is unlimited storage available for excess fat. When the adipocytes or fat cells get full, new ones form. Therefore, take steps to consume 20 to 25 percent of your total energy intake as fat. Of that, less than 10 percent should be in the form of saturated fat. That's the type of fat that's solid at room temperature and often associated with meat products, butter and lard. Replace them with plant oils if you can. Finally, don't forget about the essential fatty acids. The average adult man needs 14 to 17 grams per day of linoleic acid, while a woman needs 11 to 12 grams per day. Linoleic acid is an Omega-6 fatty acid. This represents about 5 to 10 percent of total energy intake. Alpha-linolenic acid is an omega-3 fatty acid. Men need 1.6 grams and women 1.2 grams per day for 0.6 to 1.2 percent of total energy. These fatty acids are an integral part of cell membranes.

Sugars are found naturally in many foods, especially in the form of fructose, which is found in fruits and lactose which is found in milk. You need it, but as with fat, not the amounts you are exposed to while consuming a western diet. The pleasant taste is the primary reason that sugar is often added to otherwise bland foods. Some, such as doughnuts and cakes are made with unhealthful fats as well. Keep in mind that excess sugar will be stored as fat.

Microbiota. When I see people in my midst, I don't necessarily perceive humans. I imagine a teeming mass of 100 trillion microorganisms. Bacteria make up 90 percent of all the cells within us. That's right. We are only 10 percent human. It's perhaps more accurate to view the body as a metaphorical coral reef; an ecosystem comprised of many different species, which when in balance maintain a commensurate or even symbiotic relationship with each other. However, when the balance is thrown off, everything from depression to obesity may result. We've long known that gut bacteria produce enzymes that assist in the breakdown and absorption of some foods. They are also a source of essential vitamins, such as vitamin K, and assist with the degradation of some food-associated, cancer causing chemicals. What was not expected was the discovery of a link between certain bacteria and susceptibility to obesity, inflammation, and type 2 diabetes, each of which can impact the others. Scientists are currently at the point of experimenting with different types of pre- and probiotics to determine what the bacteria within us need. Probiotics are foods such as yogurt, which contain bacteria and thereby increase the number in the gut. Prebiotics are foods such as fiber not digested in the intestine, but utilized by the gut bacteria. What is not clear is whether it's better to have large amounts of certain bacteria, an appropriate ratio of different ones, or a large variety. It won't be long before we find out because there's a lot of research being carried out in order to answer these and other pertinent questions. At a recent Psychoneuroimmunology Research Society meeting, about one third of the research being presented addressed the role of the microbiome in modulating the brain and immune system. There are even more being presented at comparable nutrition gatherings.

Take Control of Appetite Triggers

During the Stone Age, there was no need for elaborate mechanisms to dampen hunger. A few emerged; however, they take time to signal the brain. The fact is, our ancestors didn't need natural signal to stop eating because the most effective of all was already on the scene. Food scarcity was a natural braking system in the days before fast food restaurants, refrigerators, and grocery stores. When the ground was frozen, plant foods were unavailable, and even animal sources were limited. In addition, we had to compete with other alpha animals, many of which viewed us as a source of nourishment much as we did them. Not only did our ancestors have to venture into a potentially hostile environment to acquire nutrients, but they had to expend a lot of energy tracking down the game. Therefore, it was necessary for the body to develop some powerful motivators to venture out, as well as to keep on eating when they did get lucky. These are some of those appetite regulators.

Mind the orexigenic circuit. When trying to lose weight, some foods may be your worst enemy, especially fat. That's because residing deep in your brain are the orexigenic peptides. The major players are galanin, dynorphin, enkephalin, and orexin. You may not know their names, but I'm sure you've experienced their actions. These are the chemicals that stimulate your desire to consume fatty foods. From the standpoint of energy, it makes sense. Fat packs 9 calories per gram of weight compared with 4 calories for the other two macronutrients, protein and carbohydrate. Here's the problem; these triggers of fat-craving keep going up even after you pop that piece of fried chicken into your mouth. Scientists refer to this as positive-feedback. It's the opposite of how most chemicals in the body are controlled. For example, when the reproductive hormones, estrogen and progesterone rise, that increase signals cells in the brain to turn off production. A clinical application of this principal is the birth control pill. The idea is to flood the body with artificial forms of these steroids in order to shut down the natural sequence required for ovulation. Calcium, which is critical for a multitude of bodily functions, is likewise under this type of negative-feedback control. But there are a few systems that march to the beat of their own drummer. One of them includes the hormone, oxytocin. This is the brain chemical which triggers milk-letdown in nursing mothers. Rising levels induce the release of even more. That's how the orexigenic peptides are controlled. As blood lipids, especially triglycerides start to rise after you ingest that first bite of fat, you produce greater amounts of galanin and your desire to eat fat soars. It becomes a vicious circle whereby with increased intake of fat, you produce more of the peptides that trigger the desire for even more. Whether the marketers at Lays Potato Chips understood the science is not clear. But they sure got it right when they challenged the public with the "Bet you can't eat just one!" advertising campaign.

This all makes sense from an historical perspective. Imagine it is late fall and there's a chill to the air. The villagers have succeeded in killing a large mammoth. While there might have been some limited ways to pre-serve the fat strewn red meat, they would be no match for the body's unlimited capacity to store fat in the form of adipose tissue. Therefore, better stuff as many calories as possible into the body's storage cells because there may not be another opportunity to eat like this until the spring.

There's more to it. Galanin is an antagonist of Sub-stance P, the chemical, which is responsible for the sen-sation of pain. Therefore, eating fat could help reduce some of the discomfort in those suffering from chronic pain. It's also capable of reducing the metabolism of sero-tonin. Some forms of depression are thought to be due to a reduction in brain serotonin. Therefore, by slowing the breakdown of this neurotransmitter, galanin would func-tion in much the same way that antidepressants such as Prozac and Zoloft work. As if that isn't enough, the pep-tides that increase our desire to eat fat also make us feel pretty darn good. The reward chemical is called dopa-mine and when it rises in a brain region call the nucleus accumbens, it makes you feel wonderful. Indeed, that's where cocaine, alcohol and other drugs of abuse seem to work. No wonder fatty foods are referred to as comfort foods; they taste good, improve mood, reduce pain, and activate the brain's pleasure centers!

It's OK to eat fat; you need it. The problem is scar-city is no longer a factor in those countries where obe-sity has become epidemic. We have to rely on signals coming from the brain, but they aren't all that effective in a culture of excess. We no longer face the risks our ancestors did. About the only danger is tripping on a rug while making your way to the refrigerator. And if that's a concern, then press seven buttons on your telephone and have a super-deluxe pizza delivered to your door. The problem isn't fat; rather the amounts we consume, which often far exceed what's needed. It won't be easy, but here are some steps you can take to keep from getting carried away.

Eat fat only as part of a meal, not alone as a snack. As part of a meal, there will be other foods on the plate to soften the blow, especially if fiber is included. Fiber provides the bulk necessary to start the appetite dampening signals. In addition, by attaching itself to some nutrients, fiber can slow down their absorption and in some cases carry them right on through the digestive system without their ever getting into the body.

Be Aware. A primary purpose of science is to predict. By understanding the relationship between various systems in the body and the outcomes they influence, it becomes possible to predict what is likely to happen under different scenarios. While it will be exceedingly difficult to take control over the powerful appetite driving chemicals in the brain, just knowing they exist and then understanding how they function can be an important first step in taking control. At the very least, you've learned the situations to avoid. For example, don't snack on potato chips or any type of fatty foods. Grab a piece of fruit. Or if you can't resist the dip, at least scoop it up with a piece of celery, not bread. The fiber may help slow the absorption of the fat thereby reducing the probability of triggering the orexigenic peptide circuit.

Watch the alcohol. Both acute and chronic alcohol consumption can stimulate dynorphin release. That's one of the peptides capable of triggering the desire to eat more fat. In turn, the consumption of fat has been found to increase the desire for alcohol. No wonder Super Bowl Sunday is the day when both the most fat and alcohol are consumed in the United States. This is relevant for two reasons; while fat contains the most calories at 9 per gram, alcohol runs a close second at 7 per gram. That means a 12 ounce can of beer and a 6-ounce glass of wine each contain about 150 Calories. Understanding the relationship between fat and alcohol consumption will make it easier to not mix the two if your goal is to lose weight.

Ghrelin is a protein that is produced in the stomach and functions to regulate eating behavior. High levels motivate you to eat, while low levels take away that motivation by stimulating satiety centers in the brain. In other words, high levels make you hungry and low levels make you feel full. Highest levels of ghrelin are observed prior to a meal, and then drop within about an hour afterwards. Unfortunately for those attempting to lose weight, the protein increases following weight loss, which is undoubtedly one of several reasons why it's so difficult to keep the weight off after a diet.

On the other hand, some people may experience a temporal pattern of ghrelin such that if they eat at a regular time, the drop in this protein occurs within an hour after they normally eat even if they skipped the meal. It seems that a drop in this appetite triggering protein is conditioned to the time of day. Why not? If gastric secretion release can be stimulated by environmental cues, for example, the ringing of Pavlov's bell, why not other components of digestion? That means if you can resist the desire to eat long enough, your hunger may dissipate once you reach the time when the meal would normally end. If the drop in ghrelin is triggered by the time of day, why not take control of it in other ways?

Classical Conditioning

Normally, ghrelin increases as time passes since your last meal, then declines within about an hour after you finish. There's a way to keep it from going up and to speed its decline.

If you eat breakfast, lunch, and dinner at the same time each day, chances are you have conditioned the release of gastric secretions to that time of day. Or perhaps you read the newspaper with breakfast in which case retrieving it from the sidewalk becomes the trigger of appetite inducing chemicals because that's what routinely follows. If you are trying to lose weight, you don't want ghrelin whispering 'feed me' in your brains appetite centers. In order to reduce or perhaps even eliminate these automatic triggers, shuffle mealtimes so they don't occur at the same time. Part of the definition of Classical Conditioning is the fact that it can be deconditioned by breaking the association. That's exactly what you'll be doing when you start changing your mealtime. You could take this one step further and graze. Instead of eating three square meals a day, spread the number of calories you need on a daily basis over the entire day. In other words, lots of snack sized meals. Be careful. You still need nourishing foods that will provide the essential nutrients your body requires, not junk food. Just vary the time to avoid a conditioned rise in ghrelin synchronized by the clock. Let's take this one step further.

Knowing that ghrelin normally declines following a meal, start associating the digestion-induced drop with something you can control. Theoretically, anything will work. It could be an auditory cue such as a selection of music, something visual, or even an aroma. The idea is to train your GI system to automatically associate the drop in ghrelin with the cue. My recommendation is to use a pleasant odor. There are several reasons I would encourage this. First, there is already a built in connection between the sense of smell and food. That's quite evident when you have a stuffed up nose while battling a cold and realize you have lost your sense of taste. Without taste, you cannot enjoy food. And don't forget, it was both the sight and smell of meat that enticed Pavlov's dogs to salivate. It makes sense to use a sensory trigger that is already closely associated with food.

Number 2, the sense of smell, more than any other, is very closely associated with memory. It's not uncommon for a person to detect a few olfactory molecules associated with a past experience and be almost instantly transported in space and time to the place where it happened. It might be the smell of baking bread eliciting the memory of standing in their grandmother's kitchen. Or perhaps a certain fragrance that evokes the memory of their high school prom date. Conditioning is a form of subconscious memory. Your brain learns to associate something with a particular outcome, and then remembers to evoke the same response over and over. Therefore, your chances of success are much better if you select an olfactory cue to trigger a drop in ghrelin.

Number 3, compared with an auditory cue, an olfactory trigger is less intrusive. Imagine how unpopular you'd be if you started ringing a bell or blasting away on a whistle at a dinner party! There are plenty of scents to choose from. They can be found associated with candles, or special oils used in aromatherapy. Pick one you find pleasant and start experiencing it when you reach the point in a meal when your appetite begins to wane. It's doubtful the scent alone will shut off your appetite. However, by combining that sensation with other strategies, you will certainly increase your chances of success.

There's also a way you can use this strategy to block your appetite for certain categories of food. In 1967, I rode my bicycle the length of the Baja California peninsula from Tijuana to Cabo San Lucas. It was about 1000 miles through mostly desert terrain with nothing more than a deeply rutted trail for most of the ride. I was by myself and so had to carry everything I might need on the bike. World War II surplus K and C rations provided the bulk of my nourishment, and whenever I came to a ranch or settlement, I would stock up on as many calories I could before pushing on. Water was also in short supply, so I had no choice but to drink it, and in whatever form I found it when I happened upon a source. About half-way into the month long ride, I started experiencing GI symptoms, which were undoubtedly triggered by a food or water borne virus or bacteria. Who knows, perhaps a parasite as well. It wasn't until I returned to civilization and was able to drink chlorinated water that the symptoms abated. In the meantime, I suffered miserably for several weeks while pedaling my bike across the rough terrain. Needless to say, I lost my appetite for all Mexican food, especially tortillas and refried beans, which had become my staple. But then something very interesting happened. Weeks later when I decided to enjoy a dinner of Mexican food, I began to feel queasy. That put me off that category of food for several months and when I reluctantly sampled some south of the border cuisine at a party, had a similar reaction. I was experiencing what's called a conditioned aversion to the specific food my body had come to associate with the symptoms. I'm not suggesting you deliberately contaminate fatty desserts to discourage choosing them. It's just another example of how the mind can influence not only our choices of food, but through conditioning can even trigger the physiological response once experienced following exposure to illness. Your task, then, is to explore ways to mind what you eat, but in ways that will help you reach your goal.

There are other chemicals involved with regulating appetite, which may also be subject to conditioning.

Peptide YY. Countering the appetite stimulating effect of ghrelin is peptide YY, which is also produced in the gastrointestinal system. It is released after a meal and in proportion to the energy content of the food. However, when obese people finish a meal, peptide YY is produced in lesser amounts compared with a non-obese person.

Leptin is another appetite modulating hormone, but one produced by fat or adipose cells. Like peptide YY, its job is to curb eating and thereby bring about a drop in body fat. Whereas obese people still respond to the effects of ghrelin, they stop responding to leptin. It's as though they lose their sensitivity in a manner not unlike a type 2 diabetic losing sensitivity to insulin.

Uncoupling Proteins. It is deep within the cell's mitochondria where the ultimate form of energy, ATP, is produced. Glucose is eventually transported from blood into individual cells, where it is converted into ATP which fuels cellular metabolism. However, uncoupling proteins interfere with ATP production and instead generate heat. This is a form of energy expenditure that reduces the amount capable of being stored as fat. It is suspected that people with more of these uncoupling proteins would be more resistant to weight gain and obesity.

Satiety factors. A number of factors are capable of decreasing appetite. They include the same serotonin, which triggers a craving for carbohydrates when low, but which is capable of increasing satiety when high. The same is true of cholecystokinin, produced by intestinal cells. The post-meal rise in blood sugar, the expansion of the stomach walls, as well as the absorption of nutrients in the small intestines also help to curb appetite.

Appetite factor. There are a few other factors that increase appetite. The word 'endorphin' means endogenous morphine and this peptide, like its namesake, is associated with pleasure, including that resulting from eating savory food. It also increases food intake. Neuropeptide Y, not to be confused with peptide YY, is a brain peptide, which also increases appetite, especially for carbohydrate. And just as a rise in blood glucose can curb appetite, a drop in blood sugar has the opposite effect. Here are some ways you can take control in a more direct way.

Optimize Pleasure

We all need pleasure. It can be obtained in many ways including intimacy, listening to your favorite music, exercise, socializing, as well as eating tasty foods. When you are experiencing an abnormally high amount of stress, finding time to seek pleasure is going to be a challenge. But there's one thing you must make time for and that's eating, so make the most of each meal by extracting all the pleasure you can. Do the following:

a. **Slow down when eating.** Prolong the pleasure. There won't be time for that if you hurriedly shovel what's on your plate into your mouth in record time. Allow time for the food molecules to linger at the taste receptors in your mouth so you maximize the pleasant sensation.

b. **Minimize the amount of food you put on your fork.** Spread out the pleasure. In addition, there are enzymes in saliva that start breaking down carbohydrates. However, they are quickly inactivated by the acid in your stomach. It will help your digestion to allow them time to get things started.

c. **Select tasty food.** When a person eats a meal they describe as tasting so-so, they will eat over 20 percent more compared with eating the same entrée, but prepared in a way they describe as being delicious. It seems as though your brain is expecting to get some pleasure out of the dining experience and if it doesn't get it, you'll keep eating until it does.

Optimize the Natural Brakes

A number of chemicals will prompt you to either eat or stop. Other chemicals turn your appetite off, but not unless you allow them time to signal the brain that you've had enough. You can take control of these by doing the following:

d. **Snack before dinner.** Have an apple or other piece of fruit 10 minutes before sitting down at the table. It's comprised mostly of water and fiber so is bulky. Neither of those nutrients is converted into calories, however, the bulk will fool receptors in the stomach into thinking you've just finished dinner. That will create the illusion you don't need to eat as much.

e. **Slow down when eating.** In addition to the benefits described previously, slowing down will allow time for the chemicals that tell you, "Stop eating," to make their way to the brain. There are several that do this, but it's not instantaneous. If you eat too fast, you'll override these signals and when they eventually do arrive, it's too late; you've already consumed considerably more than you needed, and when the indigestion sets in, more than you wanted.

f. **Pay attention to needs.** Many people eat what they want instead of what they need. When you reach the point during a meal when you want seconds or thirds, but could leave the table and be OK, push the plate away. Many people do the opposite. They eat what they want, not what they need. Using this approach instead of sticking to the same daily calorie count will allow flexibility. For example, you may need to eat more after a day of mowing the lawn or shoveling the car from a snow drift.

g. **Eat dessert.** That's right. Have some dessert. However, not 'death by chocolate' or a bowl of ice cream. A piece of fruit or just a cup of tea will do the trick. There are two reasons for doing this. First, it will be easier to push the entry plate away when you know there's something else coming, and you'll cap the meal off with something pleasurable.

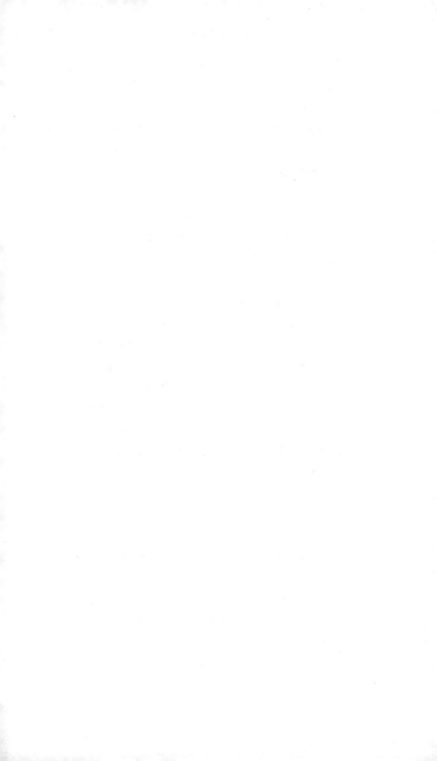

Summary Guidelines

Y ou need to eat a certain number of food calories per day to remain healthy, not just to meet your energy needs, but also to receive the vitamins and minerals your organs must have. And while you're at it, it would be a good idea to cut back on those foods capable of causing harm. It may seem daunting, but it really isn't if you simply listen to your body and follow these guidelines. They will help you manage your body weight in the most healthful way possible and should be applied at all stages of the process you engage to better manage body weight.

These are the dietary guidelines taken directly from the USDA Dietary Guidelines for Americans.

Foods and Food Components to Reduce
- *Reduce daily sodium intake to less than 2,300 milligrams (mg) and further reduce intake to 1,500*

mg among persons if you are 51 and older and those of any age who are African American or have hypertension, diabetes, or chronic kidney disease. The 1,500 mg recommendation applies to about half of the U.S. population, including children, and the majority of adults.

- *Consume less than 10 percent of calories from saturated fatty acids by replacing them with monounsaturated and polyunsaturated fatty acids.*

- *Consume less than 300 mg per day of dietary cholesterol.*

- *Keep trans fatty acid consumption as low as possible by limiting foods that contain synthetic sources of trans fats, such as partially hydrogenated oils, and by limiting other solid fats.*

- *Reduce the intake of calories from solid fats and added sugars.*

- *Limit the consumption of foods that contain refined grains, especially refined grain foods that contain solid fats, added sugars, and sodium.*

- *If alcohol is consumed, it should be consumed in moderation—up to one drink per day for women and two drinks per day for men—and only by adults of legal drinking age.*

Foods and Nutrients to Increase

Individuals should meet the following recommendations as part of a healthy eating pattern while staying within their calorie needs.

- *Increase vegetable and fruit intake.*
- *Eat a variety of vegetables, especially dark-green and red and orange vegetables and beans and peas.*
- *Consume at least half of all grains as whole grains. Increase whole-grain intake by replacing refined grains with whole grains.*
- *Increase intake of fat-free or low-fat milk and milk products, such as milk, yogurt, cheese, or fortified soy beverages.*
- *Choose a variety of protein foods, which include seafood, lean meat and poultry, eggs, beans and peas, soy products, and unsalted nuts and seeds.*
- *Increase the amount and variety of seafood consumed by choosing seafood in place of some meat and poultry.*
- *Replace protein foods that are higher in solid fats with choices that are lower in solid fats and calories and/or are sources of oils.*
- *Use oils to replace solid fats where possible.*
- *Choose foods that provide more potassium, dietary fiber, calcium, and vitamin D, which are nutrients of concern in American diets. These foods include vegetables, fruits, whole grains, and milk and milk products.*

The Art of Eating

've included a lot of science in this book, because I believe that when you understand how a particular recommendation works, it becomes easier to embrace. However, you should never allow the science of nutrition to interfere with the art of eating. There are very few pleasures left that are still legal, and eating tasty foods happens to be one of them. And one of the most enjoyable is dining out with friends. You can continue to do that despite the fact a Chef's goal is to entertain, not make you healthy. There is a way you can dine out and avoid demolishing your weight management program. Here are some suggestions:

- Avoid all-you-can-eat buffets.
- Order your meal from the children's menu or split a regular entrée with a friend.
- Instead of an entrée, consider an appetizer as your main course. But avoid those that are breaded, fried or filled with cheese.

- Select a broth-based soup instead of one that is cream-based.
- Order a lean-cut beef, fish, or poultry burger and request it be broiled or grilled instead of fried or breaded.
- Avoid dishes with cream sauces and cheese.
- Use low-fat or nonfat dressing on the side, then dip your fork in it between bites, instead of pouring it onto the salad. You'll get the flavor with every bite and significantly reduce the calories.
- Choose baked potatoes instead of mashed potatoes or rice. Even better would be substituting steamed vegetables.
- Select a low calorie beverage, such as water, or tea. Avoid soda, but if you must, make a diet version.
- Don't skip dessert, instead share one with friends or order fresh fruit.

Whether you are dining at home or eating out, always focus upon eating

- Slow down not only to allow satiety signals to reach the brain and prevent you from eating too much, but also to prolong your exposure to the pleasant flavors.
- Take small bites and make yourself aware of all the sensations arising from the food, not just the taste. Develop an awareness of the texture, aroma, and temperature as well.
- If you are with someone, conversing during the meal will result in regular pauses between bites,

which will help prolong the pleasure. If alone, make it a point to wait a few seconds between bites.

- Avoid distractions such a TV or messages on your smart phone. They will divert your attention from enjoying the meal.

Wrap It Up

It should be readily apparent that losing body weight is a formidable task. Everything from what your mother ate when she became pregnant, your experiences as a child, and the amount of stress you're experiencing as an adult are factors capable of tipping the scales toward success or failure. Add on the TV commercials enticing you to buy a pizza, the convenience of cheap, ready to go meals at the local drive-thru window, and the possibility that someone else in the family does the shopping and you may give up before even starting. However, I firmly believe that the first step toward success is an awareness of what you're up against. That knowledge provides the ability to predict, which lessens the fear you'll fail. You've known what to do, and now you have the tools to achieve the success you so richly deserve.

Note from the Author

Thank you for reading *I Know How to Lose Weight, So Why Can't I Keep It Off?* In this book, we have been exploring why this question is so common among all of us "mere mortals" who have struggled with weight issues throughout our lives. You may be asking, who is Nick Hall? And why is he qualified to teach me about such an important topic like weight loss? Let me give you a bit of my background as it relates to this topic.

After spending two years researching stress-related communication patterns in whales and dolphins for the Office of Naval Research, I went to graduate school where I completed studies in Neuroscience and then post-doctoral training in Immunology. I then spent the better part of 30 years researching the chemical pathways linking the brain with the immune system. The field is called Psychoneuroimmunology and over the years my NIH funded research ran the gambit from assessing the use of guided imagery in cancer patients, to how malnutrition and exercise impact the brain and immune system. I now spend most of my time applying this research with elite athletes and corporate clients at the Saddlebrook Resort Wellness Center, which I direct. I also teach Human Nutrition at the University of South Florida College of Nursing.

Throughout this book, I have shared a few personal experiences as examples of the information presented to you. During part of July and August in 2015 I conducted a 3,000 mile unsupported solo bicycle ride across the United States to raise money in support of Rotary International's End-Polio campaign. During that month-long trek, I was reminded countless times of the ways food can impact sleep and mood, along with the strategies to push on despite record high temperatures in the southwestern states. As a result of experiences like this, the information I present is grounded in science, and tempered with pragmatism as I explain how you can use a basic understanding of stress and nutrition to not just lose weight, but to keep it off.

And now, after reading this book, I hope you find it will be time to take action.

CPSIA information can be obtained
at www.ICGtesting.com
Printed in the USA
BVHW040812230119
538379BV00025B/272/P

9 781722 500146